MW00756348

LeBootCamp
DIET

LeBootCamp
DIET

THE SCIENTIFICALLY PROVEN FRENCH
METHOD TO EAT WELL, LOSE WEIGHT,
AND KEEP IT OFF FOR GOOD

VALÉRIE ORSONI

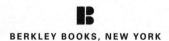

BERKLEY BOOKS, NEW YORK

THE BERKLEY PUBLISHING GROUP
Published by the Penguin Group
Penguin Group (USA) LLC
375 Hudson Street, New York, New York 10014

USA • Canada • UK • Ireland • Australia • New Zealand • India • South Africa • China

penguin.com

A Penguin Random House Company

This book is an original publication of The Berkley Publishing Group.

Library of Congress Cataloging-in-Publication Data

Orsoni, Valérie.
 Lebootcamp diet : the scientifically proven French method to eat well, lose weight, and keep it off for good / Valérie Orsoni.
  p. cm.
 ISBN 978-0-425-28060-7 (hardback)
 1. Reducing diets. 2. Reducing diets—Recipes. 3. Cooking, French. 4. Weight loss. I. Title.
 RM222.2.O82. 2015
 613.2'5—dc23
                2014048050

First edition: April 2015

PRINTED IN THE UNITED STATES OF AMERICA

10 9 8 7 6 5 4 3 2 1

Interior text design by Pauline Neuwirth.

To my son, Baptiste, for his motto:

"If there is no solution there is no problem."

So true.

CONTENTS

BOOSTER

MAINTENANCE

FOREWORD

Ms. Orsoni comes to the rescue with yet another insightful book on healthy eating and living. She does so with her constant presence of charm, wit, and positive mental attitude.

Obesity and the general degradation of healthy lifestyle has been one of the greatest challenges in medicine over the last twenty-five years. As a society, we are getting heavier, and our busy lifestyles are exposing us to the unhealthy ingredients in meals prepared outside the home. The added weight we carry is increasing our risk of a host of medical problems, from liver disease to cancers.

I have read many diet books and tried many programs, as these proliferate like bunnies in a carrot patch. This book is different in several important ways. First, Ms. Orsoni understands the importance of gradual weight loss. Rapid weight loss can result in nutritional deficiencies and unexpected new medical problems such as gallstones and inflammation in the liver. The gradual and stair-step approach in this book minimizes these risks. This approach also allows for a program of sustainable weight; the changes readers will be making are healthy habits that will benefit them over a lifetime. The best part: We can achieve health and weight loss without deprivation, enjoying delicious food in a healthful way.

Unlike fad diets, *LeBootCamp Diet*, with its four phases—Detox, Attack, Booster, and Maintenance—offers many health benefits beyond weight loss. Ms. Orsoni's eating plan shows us how to deliver antioxidants to our systems to help fight disease, particularly cancers. The use of antioxidants may help combat the constant DNA damage our bodies' cells are subject to from inflammation. Ms. Orsoni shows the way to both reduce some of this inflammation in the first place and, secondly, how to fight the toxic effects when it is there. This book also delves into some of the problems with modern foods. We have genetically altered foods under the guise of improved farming and production. One result has been the use of wheat with dramatically increased gluten content. Medicine is just beginning to understand the problems associated with gluten, even in people who do not have celiac disease.

LeBootCamp Diet shows us the way to good health and a happier life with food that is delicious, satisfying, and good for us.

Howard Hack, MD
Adjunct Clinical Associate Professor of Medicine
Stanford University School of Medicine
Stanford, California

LeBootCamp
DIET

INTRODUCTION

FOUR PHASES

FOUR PILLARS

FOUR PLEDGES

FOUR PRINCIPLES

Let me introduce myself.

I am a woman just like you.

I have battled with weight issues and frustrating fad diets for years.

I do not believe in a life of deprivation and yo-yo dieting.

After trying more than forty diets (Cabbage Soup, Paleo, the Pineapple Diet, low-calorie, dissociated [food combining], fasting, high-protein, and more); counting points with group meetings; feeding myself from pre-packaged food; after losing and regaining weight that eventually burst the seams of my jeans; after feeling taunted by so many failures and demoralized when I looked at myself in the mirror, I woke up one morning and decided that I had simply had enough!

Tired of nonsensical approaches, ranging from terribly restrictive menus to dangerously protein-rich diets, I decided to educate myself in order to understand my excess weight better and attack it intelligently.

To do this, I joined forces with my father, who was also overweight at the time. Together, we committed to maintaining a gourmet approach no matter what (we loved eating too much to deprive ourselves continuously—we are French, after all).

It may seem like something from the Stone Age, but our research led us to the library—this was well before the Internet had made its appearance in our homes. There, we devoured books on nutrition, fitness, even psychology! Gradually, we began to gather together and put to the test those concepts that seemed logical and healthy. Along the way we came to terms with the fact that if it had taken us years to gain weight, it would be unreasonable to attempt to lose it all in two weeks via tasteless meals and mono diets.

The results? After one year of a patchwork approach, which brought together everything that worked from each diet we researched, we had achieved our ideal weight, losing a total of 150 pounds between us, without any suffering or deprivation.

And then? My friends began asking for my help to get healthy and slim. I was burning out in a fast-paced corporate job at the time, so I decided to give greater meaning to my life and share this knowledge with millions of women like myself who were on the verge of giving up. Thus was born LeBootCamp.com.

Not being a doctor myself, I was soon facing criticism from those medical professionals who promote diet pills and supplements. Despite giving airtight explanations for the concepts I had proven, the program's blatant success appeared to mean very little when not dressed in medical jargon. Clearly, it was too late in life for me to go to medical school, so I surrounded myself with dozens of experts who knew more than me—physicians, dietitians, scientists, Olympic athletes, nutritionists, and psychologists—in order to test out my theories. These experts confirmed what my father and I had discovered, and together we set out to continuously improve and perfect our program.

Unlike those "miracle diets" that have remained unchanged since the seventies, LeBootCamp Diet evolves constantly, embracing new medical and scientific discoveries and ensuring that its techniques remain effective over the long term. We are diligent in our work: Indeed, we require that any new concept absorbed into LeBootCamp Diet be supported by at least five double-blind medical studies on a representative sample (a sample of five people is not valid!), according to serious and verifiable protocols.

We conducted a study to monitor eight hundred women who followed LeBootCamp program over a period of 6 months. The sample was divided into two groups of four hundred: the first group for a cholesterol study and the second group for a glycemia control study. After one month on the LeBootCamp program, the average weight loss for both groups—besides improvements in glycemia control and cholesterol levels—was 13 pounds. And after 6 months, the average weight lost and never regained, rose to 28 pounds.

And men?

Although I initially started my program catering only to the needs of women, I soon realized that BootCampers' male partners also liked the recipes, the stress-reduction exercises, and our fitness routines.

So, don't hesitate to share this book with your boyfriend, a male friend, or your partner. Enroll them in your program. Make them taste your new dishes; invite them to cook with (and for!) you. Very soon, you will have a slimmer partner—and your most loyal supporter!

In fact, except on the Turbo Detox Days, your family can totally eat like you, as the vast majority of recipes will appeal to all palates. No need to cook separately then. This will save you time, which you can use instead to exercise or practice yoga to reduce stress levels.

You now know why I created my healthy lifestyle program, a diet that works and that will make you feel good about yourself, that will help you reclaim your body without deprivations. Even if you have tried dozens of diets before, trust me and come and try it for yourself. I am excited to share your journey to your dream body. Let's get started!

FOUR PHASES

DETOX
To Cleanse Your Body

ATTACK
To Lose Weight

BOOSTER
To Speed Up the Process!

MAINTENANCE
To Ensure You Never Regain Lost Weight

1. DETOX

The foundation of the program. A 2-week phase, where my top 10 detoxifying foods are incorporated into balanced menus designed to nourish your body with antioxidants, eliminate toxins, and give you more energy.

► **WHAT YOU ACHIEVE:** The first pounds are shed quickly, energy is regained, skin is glowing.

► **KEY CONCEPT:** Detoxification.

2. ATTACK

Now that your body has been cleansed and the first few pounds are gone, you are ready to attack the stubborn weight that remains and reduce cellulite. This second phase lasts as long as it takes to lose 75 percent of the weight you need to shed. With my guidance, you will establish healthy life habits and learn how to balance your daily meals.

A Turbo Detox Day (TD Day) is featured every week, to promote the elimination of toxins and enhance weight loss. You will gradually integrate new foods and flavors into your diet through delicious, light recipes. During ATTACK you will find weight loss effective and motivating, allowing you to reach your ideal weight with ease.

► **WHAT YOU ACHIEVE:** Stubborn pounds are targeted, attacked, and eliminated; you lose 75 percent of the weight you want to shed; cellulite is greatly reduced; body is toned.

► **KEY CONCEPTS:** Glycemic load and its impact on weight loss. Additionally, during this phase I will introduce you to the concept of benchmarking, a strategy that ensures you continue to lose weight as you go along. You'll learn how to transform those dreaded "plateaus" into secure milestones, each one a personal victory.

3. BOOSTER

This enhancing routine lasts 7 days and recurs several times throughout the program. You should repeat it every time you reach the end of a benchmark during the ATTACK phase or, once you are in the MAINTENANCE phase, whenever you feel the need to renew yourself; for example, after a girls' weekend, after a holiday where the food was plentiful and irresistible, after a period of intense stress at work, or if you are keen to achieve a flatter stomach. This short phase will also help you gain a flat stomach thanks to the latest studies and discoveries in gut health. We will explore how certain foods can increase the level of our candida, thereby leading to bloating and pain. Conversely, we will help you identify which foods can help reduce this problem, thereby helping you get the flat tummy of your dreams.

Throughout these short intervals, we abstain from meat, dairy, yeast, gluten, and alcohol in order to truly support the detoxifying functions of our body.

► **WHAT YOU ACHIEVE:** A cleansed body more able to lose pounds quickly, and a flat abdomen.

► **KEY CONCEPTS:** Intense cleansing and the yeast connection.

4. MAINTENANCE

This last phase is unlimited. With the help of this book, and also with our Facebook page (facebook.com/groups/lebootcampdiet) and its active community; our website (LeBootCamp.com); and our Twitter and Instagram feeds (twitter.com/valerieorsoni; @valerieorsoni), you will learn to create balanced menus for yourself as well as handle various life challenges: restaurants, parties, social engagements, traveling, and so on.

Once you have shed your final pounds, your weight will naturally stabilize. Physical activity will become an integral part of your daily life as you tone those last few stubborn areas. By then you will know how to avoid nutritional pitfalls and the trap of fad diets. You will be ready to pursue your healthy journey independently and with confidence, and will never regain your lost weight!

▶ **WHAT YOU ACHIEVE:** Your ideal weight is maintained and your energy levels are high. You love your body!

▶ **KEY CONCEPT:** Alkaline-balancing to support a healthy life and keep the pounds off.

FOUR PILLARS

1. GOURMET NUTRITION

Some eat to live. I live to eat, and personally, I am convinced that there is nothing worse than a life governed by deprivation and tasteless meals. Yes, I promise you, we can live a healthy, long life AND enjoy delicious foods from all food groups.

Back when I was a child growing up in France, my dad was a chef and I had the privilege of being introduced to a cuisine rich in diversity that shaped my taste buds—though, I must admit, there are foods I cannot even imagine myself eating anymore (think snails or tripe). Let's go back to our roots, when we truly enjoyed everything that nature has to offer. There are no forbidden foods in my program!

2. EASY FITNESS

Let's face it, we all have hectic lives and rarely use our gym membership (that is, if we can afford one in the first place). We need to reclaim our birthright and rediscover what our bodies were designed to do when we were fit and trim without the gym. There is a direct correlation between the advent of gyms, food labels, new diets, and obesity, and it is not what we think. The obesity epidemic did not, in fact, give rise to these. Shockingly, it is the reverse. By infantilizing society, these familiar props of modern life have only worsened the problem.

In truth, in our most natural state, we shouldn't have to suffer, military style, to get in shape, or force ourselves to sweat for hours at the gym. This is precisely what the fitness aspect of my program is about: getting your heart pumping and your muscles moving without too much effort—the "in-shape-no-sweat" approach. Follow my "25th-hour" exercises (pages 42–46) and you'll see how easy it is to fit exercise into an already busy day.

3. MOTIVATION

Knowing what's right is not enough. The proof? Hundreds of books have been published on health and dieting by doctors, gurus, nutritionists, nurses, dietitians, and coaches—yet still, nobody has succeeded in reducing the obesity epidemic.

On the other hand, learning what works one day at a time, while incorporating small but effective new techniques, is the surest path to a slimmer you. A study conducted at the University of California–Berkeley proved this fact beyond any doubt. Two groups of individuals were observed over the course of 18 months: the first one was given all the instructions to lose weight in one "sitting," while the second was given one element per day for 90 days. After 18 months, the second group had lost twice as much weight and kept it off for longer than the first group.

This is why I can guarantee that, if you follow my program, you will win the fight against those stubborn pounds one day at a time, step by step, until you reach your perfect weight. For the days when you feel down, when "motivation" is a meaningless word to you, when diet saboteurs challenge your grit, I will arm you with proven techniques to help you stay on track, no matter what.

4. STRESS AND SLEEP MANAGEMENT

Despite multiple studies linking stress to obesity, the connection is commonly overlooked and causes many diets to fail. Since a happy dieter is a successful dieter, I offer you a guilt-free approach, based on proven strategies that will help you reclaim your inner peace and lessen your stress levels. This will, in turn, reduce your cortisol levels, improve the quality of your sleep, and trim down belly fat. Focused exercise, abdominal breathing, visualization techniques, and my own widely-respected motivational methodologies will bring your body and mind into closer harmony. Your energy will soar.

FOUR PLEDGES

1. ETHICS

Because of my own negative experience with fad diets and simply because of the way I am wired, my approach is underpinned by the highest level of respect for you. You can trust that I abide by a strict code of ethics, in that everything I share with you is based on solid medical and scientific foundations. I've tried to present these principles in a fun way, to make them easier to understand and implement in your everyday life.

2. HEALTH

Everything we do in life should have a positive impact on our health and well-being. That's why my most fundamental objective is to enhance your fitness and vitality. After risking my own health with dangerous diets, I am now totally committed to a healthy lifestyle. And this is what I share with you in my program, firm in the belief that a healthy body is one that sheds pounds faster *(faster as in when your body is all in balance the pounds will melt off more easily than if your body is toxic)* and does not regain lost weight.

3. QUALITY

I'll be brief: Quality goes hand-in-hand with the highest standards of ethics and health; I will never compromise these standards. I am dedicated to making sure that the products and services I present to you are always of the highest degree of excellence. Enough said.

4. INNOVATION

Boredom and monotony are largely responsible when it comes to diet failures. Just take one look at how short-lived high-protein and mono diets turn out to be. I love exploring new foods, new concepts, or new fitness trends, which keep me on my toes and always on the lookout. Count on me for sharing new products and ideas with you that will make your weight-loss journey easier and more fun.

To stay informed of all my new products and concepts, check my blog regularly at www.valerieorsoni.com.

FOUR PRINCIPLES

1. NO FORBIDDEN FOOD GROUPS

▶ **FACT:** Banning certain foods leads to yo-yo dieting.

Because I have experienced firsthand what happens when you're deprived of certain foods, I made a promise to myself never, ever to inflict such extreme measures on my body again. Besides being unhealthy, this deprivation leads to obsessive-compulsive behaviors, which, in turn, trigger "yo-yo" dieting (lose weight, regain more, lose more, regain more, and so on).

Hence, no food group is banned from my diet. Some foods are evidently healthier than others—I recommend you avoid unnecessary toxins by eating organic as much as possible—and we will focus on them.

2. BODY-CLEANSING

▶ **FACT:** A clean body is a lean body. A clean body supports rapid, healthy weight loss.

Our body certainly has the right equipment to rid itself of the toxins we produce, ingest, inhale, or absorb through our skin. However, in our fast-paced world with increased environmental pollution, the rise of pesticides and other chemicals in our food chain, and the extremely high levels of stress we face, our bodies are under too much strain for basic detoxification functions to be sufficient. Hence a DETOX phase, a Turbo Detox Day (TD Day), and a recurring BOOSTER phase to support the body's cleansing ability.

3. ALKALINE-BALANCING

▶ **FACT:** An acidic body is a tired and vulnerable body. An alkaline body is an energetic and healthy body.

We measure the acidity level of our system using pH-grading, aiming for a perfect urine pH of 7 (that of pure water) to best support all our bodily functions. Most important, the rate of our weight loss improves when our body has the perfect alkaline-acid balance.

4. SUGAR MANAGEMENT

▶ **FACT:** We all consume too much refined sugar.

A direct link has been established between the rise in obesity and the dramatic rise in sugar consumption (from 10 pounds per person per year in 1815, to 120 pounds in 2000). On top of pure sugar, we consume way too many high-glycemic foods, which turn our body into fat-storing machines. Together we will learn how to enjoy the sweetness in life without jeopardizing our weight-loss efforts.

DOES MY APPROACH WORK?

Don't take my word for it! BootCampers from around the world have endorsed it. Check out their testimonials here: lebootcamp.com/testimonials.

Before letting you dive into the last diet of your life, let me also share with you the story of Patricia, my first-ever weight-loss client. It was exactly one week after Thanksgiving 2003 when I launched my online weight-loss coaching website. As much as I had mastered subjects like nutrition, fitness, and coaching, I was a total beginner when it came to business: I had no business plan, no business bank account, nor any idea of the price at which I would set my services. Let's face it: I had launched my business without thinking at all about its structure—so full of joy and hope was I at the prospect of helping other women around the world reach their ideal weight!

I was riding the Caltrain, which links San Francisco to the suburbs. A rather plump woman next to me struck up conversation.

"Gosh, you're lucky to be so skinny!" she said. "Mother Nature has been kind to you. You look amazing!" To which I replied, "Mother Nature is kind only if you help her. Trust me, I waged a battle against unwanted pounds for as long as I can remember, until I worked out a healthy strategy to get the results I'd wanted for so long. Now, I am actually launching my very own healthy program online."

"What a great idea!" she exclaimed. "How much does it cost and when can I get started?" This marked the beginning of a great adventure during which Patricia lost 44 pounds, which she never regained.

So, are you ready? Great! To help you get started, here are 10 steps I recommend you follow before embarking on phase one of my program: namely, DETOX.

TOP 10 PRE-DETOX STEPS

1. Decide on your weight-loss goal: Write it on a Post-it and place the note on the mirror in your bathroom as a constant reminder.

2. Involve your friends: Sharing a goal means being accountable. Social networks make your life easier when it comes to finding support. Sign up your friends in your fight against those unwanted pounds.

3. Decide on the start date: This is vital! By consciously choosing your first day, you will have taken the step that will guarantee that you get started.

4. Grocery shopping: Stock up on everything you will need for the first week (go to the menu plans on pages 58–67 to check out the menus and draw up your shopping list).

5. Get rid of temptations: Give away everything you won't be eating during the DETOX and BOOSTER phases.

6. Buy your equipment: To get the most out of my program you will need a juicer, a blender, a pedometer (or an app on your smartphone that counts steps and distance), and a pair of well-fitting walking shoes. If you don't have everything right away, don't fret! For instance, if you don't have a juicer then you can mix your fruits/veggies in a blender and strain the juice with a piece of muslin or cheesecloth.

7. Walk: Start walking for 30 minutes every single morning before your breakfast—but after your morning drinks: lemon water, green tea, and Sobacha (page 69). Get your heart pumping! (P.S. Studies show that this is most beneficial, but if you absolutely cannot walk in the mornings, do so on an empty stomach before lunch or dinner.)

8. Pre-detox: Not quite ready to start today? No problem! Get set right now by doing a few things to make sure you don't keep delaying the true start. Get going by eliminating red meat and dairy from your daily meals.

9. Drink water: Drink at least 8 glasses of water each day. Keep in mind that hydration needs vary from person to person. The best way to determine if you should drink more is to look at the color of your urine; if it is dark yellow it means you aren't drinking enough; if it's clear, you are already doing a great job.

10. Weigh yourself! Do this right now, and then once a week, if that works for you. Once you begin the DETOX phase, weigh yourself daily or at least every other day. After the DETOX phase, I suggest you stick to a time frame that works for you: If you find daily weigh-ins too stressful for you, then go for weekly weigh-ins, but never have more than 7 days in between weigh-ins to make sure you stay on track. (I personally like a daily weigh-in to stay on track.) Record your starting weight on "Your Weight-Loss Progress Page" (page 351).

WHAT IS MY IDEAL WEIGHT?

*a*LL WEIGHT-LOSS experts (me included) have tried to come up with a perfect formula. Even if it is important to know how to calculate one's ideal weight (because this will be our target), you should remember that there is no perfect solution, no magic number.

Indeed, among all the formulas dreamed up by doctors, online calculators, and insurance companies (which very often add 4 to 22 pounds to what we consider our sexy, ideal weight), it is extremely difficult to know whom to trust, especially when we are also being bombarded with images of extremely skinny models in women's magazines.

So how can we evaluate our ideal weight? Start by using the Creff formula, which calculates your ideal weight (in kilograms) purely from a health perspective. (There are many online conversion calculators you can use to convert your results; try www .onlineconversion.com.) This formula corrects the more famous Lorentz formula as it brings in two further considerations: age and morphology.

Have you ever heard someone say, "I can never be skinny because I have big bones"? Well, with the Creff formula, the size of your bones is taken into consideration. In terms of morphology, for an individual with a slight frame, 10 percent is subtracted from the weight calculated for an average person. Conversely, for someone with a large morphology, 10 percent is added to the average ideal weight.

To determine if you are small, average, or broad, place the middle finger and thumb of your right hand around your left wrist:

SMALL your thumb slightly overlaps your middle finger
AVERAGE your thumb and finger just touch
BROAD your thumb and finger don't even touch

Continued . . .

CREFF FORMULA

Small morphology:

[(height in centimeters) − 100 + (age in years/10)]
    x 0.9 x 0.9

Average morphology:

[(height in centimeters) − 100 + (age in years/10)] x 0.9

Broad morphology:

[(height in centimeters) − 100 + (age in years/10)]
    x 0.9 x 1.1

NOTE: This formula is only one indication of your health. It is totally possible that your perceived ideal weight (the one at which you feel proud of yourself in your bikini) is under (rarely over) this number. For example, my ideal weight is 8 pounds under the weight determined by the Creff formula.

It is essential to keep in mind that your ideal weight is the one you can maintain without depriving yourself and without intense efforts. For instance, I am 5 feet 3 and have a small morphology. If I weigh 106 pounds, I look hot on TV and in a bikini, but it is extremely hard for me to maintain this weight, and I need to truly deprive myself to stay at that level. I get ill easily and my energy levels are low. Now, if I use the Creff formula my ideal weight is 121 pounds, but then I feel heavy and sluggish—far from the energetic bunny I have become famous for being. However, when I am 115 pounds, I am generally at the top of my game, energy-wise, and almost never sick.

Now it is your turn to determine your ideal weight, using the Creff formula to start with, before comparing it with where you feel your best. This will be your personal "cruising weight," and the one we will be aiming to reach and maintain.

DETOX

GOAL:

DETOX YOUR LIFESTYLE

AND RESET YOUR BODY

TO LOSE YOUR FIRST

POUNDS RAPIDLY

DETOX

> ▶ **FACT:** Stress is fattening; the accumulation of toxins stemming from our lifestyle, environment, and food prevents us from losing weight.

RULES OF THE DETOX PHASE

- Detox your body with **5** detox foods per day. It is very important that even if you modify the menus, you stick to this magic number.
- Drink Sobacha every morning, plus 3 cups throughout the day. Sobacha is an infusion made with toasted buckwheat. The recipe is on page 69.
- Drink lemon juice with water every morning.
- Avoid red meat; cow dairy; eggs; rich sauces like tartar or hollandaise sauce; sugar products; heavy foods like mayonnaise, pizzas, or enchiladas; gluten; and alcohol, all of which can overload our system in different ways.
- We do 5 "25th-hour" exercises per day.
- We manage our stress with abdominal breathing exercises.

These first 14 days of my program are critical to the success of my weight-loss strategy. That is why I urge you *not* to skip directly to the second phase (I know some might be tempted). Everything has been designed to put you on the right track to a slimmer you. Thousands of women have followed my program, and it's thanks to their valuable feedback that I have been able to devise and adapt this first, vital phase.

I must warn you right away: These 2 weeks won't be the easiest in my plan. But rest assured, they remain true to my philosophy of yummy nutrition and easy fitness. If you're feeling apprehensive, just project yourself to the place, 2 weeks from now, when you'll be feeling the full effects of this detox: Your first few pounds will have vanished, leaving you feeling lighter, more energetic, and highly motivated!

WHAT IS A DETOX?

In the strict sense of the word, detoxification means helping our body get rid of addictive or toxic substances.

The word *detox* appeared for the first time in an American women's magazine in 1973—a time when our world had started spinning faster and our days were becoming more hectic: moms working but still keeping their full-time job as moms; technology that was supposed to help us be more efficient but instead blurred the lines between life and work; longer working hours; economic crises pushing individuals to work longer and harder to make ends meet; and the list goes on and on. Incidentally, that is when we also noticed a spike of overweight people in the Western world.

Forty years later, this term has broadened to cover a vast range of therapies, from the rehab of substance-abuse addicts to extreme fasts designed to flush toxins out of the system to simply abstaining from a variety of indulgences.

WHY DO TOXINS PREVENT ME FROM LOSING WEIGHT?

A toxin is a substance that our body does not need and which requires energy to be eliminated. Even some elements vital to our survival, such as certain nutrients, can become toxic in large quantities. As my grandmother used to say, "Too much of a good thing can be bad!"

Not only are we surrounded by toxins—bacteria, parasites, viruses, pesticides, pollution, and chemical products (including chemical-loaded beauty products)—but we also directly ingest a large portion of toxins via the food we eat. Thus, food becomes our number-one source of toxins! Remember that toxins can be carcinogenic, and "carcinogenic" means "can cause cancer."

The beauty of the detox process is that food, our first source of toxicity, is also the best and easiest way to clean up our body. What's more, weight loss will automatically begin as you start to detox!

How so? Our body handles toxic aggressions by encapsulating toxins in fat cells; hence, the more toxins we carry, the larger our fat cells become. The detoxification process helps reduce the area of fat mass where these fat-soluble toxins are stored.

Here's the equation: When we reduce the toxin content in our body we reduce the quantity of fat that is stored. Then we enter a virtuous circle where we have fewer toxins to store and, therefore, less fat required to store them.

HOW DOES THE BODY ELIMINATE TOXINS NATURALLY?

The word *detox*, is, unfortunately, often misused by charlatans around the world touting miracle pills and potions to cleanse the body. And it greatly antagonizes some doctors, who refuse even to acknowledge that the concept exists. They argue that the body is naturally equipped to clean itself through its hepatic and kidney functions and that detox programs serve no purpose.

However, those old-school doctors might as well go back to . . . school! You need only to look at an alcoholic's liver or the lungs of a heavy smoker to realize that even the perfectly programmed human body has its limits when it comes to getting rid of toxins. Yet there's just no need for expensive (and, sometimes, dangerous) detox products or programs. My DETOX phase is simple, proven, affordable—and it will help you shed your unwanted pounds. Trust your coach!

THE BODY HAS DEVELOPED TWO WAYS OF ELIMINATING TOXINS

1. Internal: Our body has an extraordinarily complex system that modifies, attacks, and eliminates threats to our health. For hundreds of thousands of years, the human body has been reliant upon this system. Unfortunately for us, with the drastic increase in the number of toxic products we are now exposed to, and their poor quality, our liver, stomach, immune system, kidneys, and lungs can't cope with the load anymore. So, we need to support our organs by way of a complete detox program.

2. External: Our skin can also help us eliminate a large quantity of toxins, thanks to the sweat glands. Supporting this function is very easy: You need to sweat! You can do this either by exercising, or—even more efficiently—by sitting in a steam room or sauna for a prescribed time.

> ▶ **NOTE:** Never stay longer than 20 minutes in a sauna and never use the sauna as an alternative to exercise or a healthy diet.

In our daily life, we can point the finger at three major sources of toxins that are responsible for, among other things, our extra weight: food, stress, and external pollutants. Together, we shall take action against those three culprits.

TOXIC DIETS

*e*XTREME DIETS can actually be a source of toxins. If you have ever followed a high-protein diet, you have most likely regained all the weight you lost; you might also remember that during this diet your skin looked dull, your breath was terrible, your energy low, your mood swings extreme, and your headaches frequent. Nutritionist associations and some followers of high-protein diets have even reported kidney failure as a direct result of this diet.

Why? Because your body is not equipped to eliminate the excessive amount of protein residues (ketone bodies) generated when exposed to a radically high protein intake. These residues are toxins that have to be eliminated through our kidneys. This is why you have to drink a lot of water on a high-protein diet.

The same toxic punishment results if you follow a mono diet like the Cabbage Soup Diet, the Pineapple Diet, or the Lemon Juice/Cayenne Pepper Diet.

And if you think that fasting will solve the problem, you are totally mistaken! In fact, pushed outside its healthy comfort zone, our fasting body will get its energy from fat stores and from our muscle mass (not from our digestive tract or glycogen reserves as in a normal, balanced diet). This leads to a high production of waste, causing an increase of the toxin levels in the body.

FOOD

Our refined modern diet is often characterized by excessive protein and a deficient fiber content, with too much saturated fat, too much sugar, and too much sodium (that's your table salt).

More than 2,800 substances (preservatives, artificial colors, sweeteners) are used by the food industry to improve taste, texture, color, and the shelf life of products. The problem is that these additives often increase the toxin levels in our body. Add to these the pesticides used to grow your food and you have an explosive mix of toxins that the body struggles to excrete, leaving it exhausted (one of the reasons you're feeling so tired!).

TOP FIVE TOXINS IN OUR FOOD

1. Mercury from Large, Carnivorous Fish

I love fish, as they are rich in healthy fats (those famous omega-3s, said to boost brain function) and lean protein. Fish possess precious nutritional qualities. The problem is that they are also contaminated by environmental pollutants like dioxins, methylmercury, PCBs (polychlorinated biphenyls), and so on. Mercury can mainly be found in fatty fish like tuna and the flesh of other wild predators in the fish family. Because they are so high up the food chain, larger fish accumulate more of those pollutants by eating smaller fish.

Chronic exposure to mercury has been proven to have terrible health consequences, notably for our nervous system, leading to tingling in the limbs, blurred vision, hearing problems, and cognitive deficiencies. Exposure to methylmercury while pregnant can also trigger neurological developmental delays and growth issues in the fetus. Furthermore, methylmercury can also have an adverse impact on our digestive system and kidneys.

For these reasons, I advise you to limit yourself to small fish such as anchovies and sardines, wild fish from protected places like Alaska (although they will still contain some environmental toxins, owing to water flowing freely around the globe), or organically farmed fish. I really insist on organic fish farming, as non-organic fish farms frequently use food with questionable ingredients, some of them very toxic. Don't take my word for it, go and visit one!

2. Pesticides and Chemical Treatments Used in Agriculture

Some environmental toxins, like chemical fertilizers, pesticides, fungicides, and other synthetic products used by the agriculture industry, can be found in the fruits and vegetables you buy at your favorite market. The problem with these toxic elements is that, once ingested, they can mimic our "body messengers," or hormones. That is why pesticides are often called "endocrine disruptors." Some pesticides are capable of mimicking the effects of estrogens—hormones produced naturally by our body—and can cause numerous illnesses such as obesity, diabetes, and cardiovascular diseases. Overexposure to estrogens has also been proven to increase the risk of breast cancer. Indeed, by affecting your endocrine system, those pesticides can affect the actions of neurotransmitters (chemical messengers, such as serotonin) and have a negative impact on your metabolism.

> ▶ **FACT:** The average Golden Delicious apple receives 32 chemical treatments from the time of pollination until its arrival on your plate. Go organic!

3. High-Fructose Corn Syrup (HFCS)

The term *fructose syrup* makes us think of ordinary white sugar, in its liquid form. However, high-fructose corn syrup is actually far from natural and is becoming increasingly common in our food. You may well be consuming it without even knowing. Check the labels on your sweets, breads, and ready-made meals. Even innocent-looking crackers may contain it. So, what is it?

This syrup, invented in 1957, is made primarily from cornstarch. Its low cost—three times less expensive than sugar—together with its superior sweetening and taste-enhancement properties, make it a perfect candidate for the manufacturing of low-priced sweets and baked goods. It's now ubiquitous on supermarket shelves and is slowly but surely replacing the traditional sucrose (ordinary white sugar) in processed foods.

Replacing sucrose with high-fructose corn syrup has little or no impact on taste. However, the effect of HFCS on our hormonal functions is an invisible menace.

But why, you might wonder, is fructose a "good" sugar when present in fruit, but not when it is found in HFCS? Fructose in fruits is okay because it is combined with fiber, water, and other ingredients. Isolated from fiber (which slows down the digestion of sugar) and consumed in large quantities, HFCS will increase our triglyceride (fat) and cholesterol levels, leading to an over-storage of fat and excess weight.

I'm sure you get the picture: In order to remain slim or to lose weight, you must become an educated shopper and always read food labels. If you see HFCS, fructose/glucose sugar, fructose/glucose syrup, corn sugar, or corn syrup on the label, don't buy it!

4. Artificial Sweeteners

I am deeply convinced that the black sheep of the dieting world is artificial sweetener. Official studies and meta-studies prove that it is largely responsible for the obesity epidemic and for the fact that the vast majority of overweight individuals find it hard to lose weight.

These sweeteners have been invading our food for decades. With a sweetening power equal or superior to that of regular white sugar, artificial sweeteners don't contain any calories. What a miracle! Finally to be able to consume sweet foods without putting on weight—who hasn't dreamed of it? So, what's the catch?

Researchers have found that if we trick our brain into thinking that we are eating something sweet without the intake of calories our body is expecting, the sweet craving is exacerbated. A study by Irish researchers looking at the impact of diet drinks on the eating habits of ordinary people (not athletes) proved this beyond doubt. They concluded that diet drinks and foods blur our ability to sense hunger.

> ▶ **FACT:** Diet foods can be a trap. They are expensive and can never replace a balanced diet.

Let's look at the most often used sweeteners on the market and you'll see that some represent a far healthier choice than others:

- **Acesulfame-K:** This synthetic sweetener has a sweetening power 200 times stronger than that of regular sugar but contains zero calories. It is highly resistant to heat, so can be used for baking.

However, it is literally too good to be true, as it can't be metabolized by the body. To be avoided.

- **Aspartame:** This artificial sweetener, also called E951, was created in 1965 and is 200 times sweeter than sugar. Since its launch on the U.S. market in 1974, it has caused a great deal of controversy but, owing to a very powerful lobby, it has succeeded in remaining in our food. It can now be found in almost all "diet" or "light" yogurts, baked goods, sweets, chewing gums, and ice cream.

Even though aspartame is calorie-free, it still affects your blood sugar levels just like white sugar would, by stimulating the pancreas to produce insulin. This reaction causes the body to store more of the "real" food you've eaten, in the form of fat.

That's why even low-calorie carbonated drinks (very likely to be sweetened with aspartame), transform you into a fat-storing machine. What's more, if the fizzy drink is served freezing cold, as is commonly the case, your appetite will be further intensified and you will most likely order more food. In terms of drinks, you are always better off with water or green tea (which has a low caffeine content).

▶ **NOTE:** In December 2013, the European Food Safety Authority published a report claiming that aspartame is safe and poses no threat to our health. It is interesting to note that in the United States this sweetener is not recommended for pregnant women or diabetics—but this is not the case in France, Italy, or the UK.

- **Erythritol:** Though discovered in 1874, it took some years before this was used by the food industry. Erythritol, a polyol, or sugar alcohol, is a natural sweetener found in fruits, fermented foods, and soy sauce. It has a slightly higher sweetening power than sugar, with two advantages: It does not cause cavities and contains zero calories. So far, no study has ever shown its danger to our health.
- **Fructose:** This natural fruit sugar has the lowest glycemic index among all the sweeteners and has long been recommended to diabetics as a sugar substitute. However, after more research, we

know that although fructose does not cause a rise in blood sugar, it does trigger an increase in triglyceride levels (fat levels in the blood). So, it's fine to consume fructose in its natural form (as the fiber contained in fruit prevents the triglyceride level increase), but it should never be used as a sweetener. To be avoided.

EFFECTS OF ASPARTAME ON APPETITE

*t*HE IMPACT of aspartame on weight gain has been proven numerous times, but one of my favorite studies is the famous one conducted by Dr. Katherine Appleton, of Queen's University, Belfast:

Three runners are given a bottle of liquid to drink, without knowing what it is.

The first bottle contains water, the second one contains a fizzy drink sweetened with ordinary sugar, and the third bottle contains a diet drink sweetened with aspartame.

After each runner has drank her bottle, she is made to run for 20 minutes.

After the run, each participant is presented with an identical meal with one instruction: Stop eating when you aren't hungry anymore.

This experiment is repeated over the course of 10 years, and the same result is noted each time: The runners eating more are always the ones who initially consumed the diet drink. On average, they take in around 150 extra calories at each meal.

Despite Katherine Appleton's research, manufacturers of diet drinks consistently deny that their products cause an increased feeling of hunger.

But if it's true that drinking a diet soda sweetened with aspartame before a meal increases your food intake by 150 calories, as Dr. Appleton concluded, after 50 days this will lead to a weight gain of around 2 pounds (since you need approximately 7,000 extra calories to make 2 pounds of fat).

Scary!

- **Maltitol:** This sweetener is responsible for that intense sense of freshness you get from some foods (notably chewing gums). Another polyol, maltitol is one of the rare sweeteners to be authorized for diabetics because it does not affect blood sugar. It is derived from maltose (found in starch) and can have laxative effects in large quantities. Unlike some other sweeteners, it is non-cavity-forming and should be chosen over aspartame. It's not calorie-free, though: It contains 2.4 calories per gram (as opposed to 4 calories per gram for sucrose).

- **Monk fruit:** A native of Thailand and China, this naturally sweet fruit has been cultivated for over 800 years. Its extract is 300 times sweeter than sugar and brings zero calories. So far very few studies have shown adverse side effects so it is deemed to be a safe natural sweetener for everyday use. Beware that as manufacturers jump on the monk-fruit-sugar bandwagon, some of the "monk fruit products" may contain ingredients like alcohol, molasses, fructose, sucrose, and others. The vast majority will contain dextrose, a carbohydrate derived from corn used here to help make the monk fruit extract edible (it is otherwise way too potent and needs to be diluted).

- **Saccharine:** The dinosaur of all artificial sweeteners! Created in 1879, it has a very high sweetening power (300 to 400 times that of regular sugar), zero calories, and leaves a strong metallic taste in the mouth. Saccharine withstands heat and has a long shelf life, so it is now used as a stabilizer in combination with other sweeteners. Because saccharine was once thought to cause cancer in humans, the FDA required manufacturers to put a warning label on products containing it. In 2000, however, the warning labels were removed, as scientists discovered that in the case of saccharine, the results of the studies done on lab rats did not apply to humans.

- **Stevia:** Consumed in Japan since the fifties, stevia now represents more than 75 percent of the sweeteners sold in this country. Although no study proving any health dangers has ever been published, it still took years for other countries to authorize stevia as a food supplement. As of 2014, it can be found in all Western countries. Stevia is a herbaceous plant from the Asteraceae family. Its leaves, dried and crushed, have a very sweet taste and have been used for thousands of years in South America and China. It has zero calories and a sweetening power 150 to 300 times higher than that of sugar. You can use stevia for baking, but not for making jams, as it cannot be heated above 400°F. Stevia also lowers blood sugar levels, reduces blood pressure, and is a natural, mild diuretic. Since it does not increase blood sugar it is a natural ally for diabetics. Recommended until proven otherwise.

- **Sucralose:** Found everywhere (except France where it was banned in 2012) and made from ordinary white sugar (sucrose). It has a high sweetening power with zero calories. Following a few studies pointing out potential dangers, it has suffered from rather bad press. However, no serious double-blind study has been conducted for long enough to gauge whether or not sucralose has any negative impact on health. Until there is evidence to the contrary, I avoid using it on a regular basis (but if I run out of stevia, this sweetener would be my second choice).

- **Xylitol:** This polyol is extracted from the bark of the birch tree. Often sold in powder form, xylitol has the same sweetening power and the same taste as ordinary white sugar but has half the calories. It has two main advantages: It protects our teeth by preventing the fermentation of bacteria and also remineralizes teeth (i.e., hardens the enamel), a property that none of the other polyols have.

5. Other Additives: Artificial Colorings, Flavor Enhancers, and Preservatives

We have been using additives since the dawn of time (well, almost) to improve taste, texture, color, and the shelf life of food. Romans used saltpeter (or potassium nitrate), Egyptians used food colorings, and toward the end of the nineteenth century, the first chemical leavening agent was created. As we've discussed, while many of these have huge advantages, they also increase the toxin levels in our body, which can lead to weight gain.

The biggest culprit is MSG (monosodium glutamate; code name E621 and also known as glutamate, sodium glutamate, glutamic acid, monopotassium glutamate, and GMS). It is truly ubiquitous and can be found in chips, "homemade" soups, sweets, and in almost all ready-made meals. However, not only does MSG contain nothing good for our body, it also increases our appetite, thus making us overeat.

It's simple: Avoid all products containing MSG and you will have made one solid step toward easy weight loss!

Before moving on, I would like to discuss some other causes of toxicity, besides what we put on our plates: toxic substances, stress, and external pollutants.

CIGARETTES, ALCOHOL, AND CAFFEINE

CIGARETTES

Smoking poisons the body; causes gray skin tone, lower lung capacity, and fatigue; and deprives you of half your vitamin C. Passive smoking harms those around you. However, one cannot fight on all fronts simultaneously. So choose your battles in an order that works for you: Lose weight first, then stop smoking, or the reverse, but not both at the same time, or you run the risk of failure. If you do smoke, the menus at the end of this chapter will help balance this dangerous addiction by supporting your body's ability to eliminate toxins.

ALCOHOL

Alcohol can actually be good for you in very small quantities—this is the famous "French paradox." It has been proven that red wine's polyphenols can guard us against cardiovascular diseases. If you drink one glass of red wine per day (two per day for men; life is unfair!) consider yourself protected. Beyond this level, wine becomes toxic. So we will be abstaining during DETOX and BOOSTER but the rest of the time you are allowed your daily glass of red. Isn't life wonderful?

CAFFEINE

Caffeine is not a poison, but if you drink too much during the day, as with many other things, you can give yourself palpitations and sleepless nights. That said, serious studies indicate that one coffee a day (enjoyed at leisure) can bring several benefits: It keeps you alert and is packed with antioxidants. Some studies have found an association between coffee consumption and decreased overall mortality as well as cardiovascular mortality, although this may not hold true for younger people who drink large amounts of coffee.

If you plan on drinking one or two small cups of coffee, may I suggest that you gradually replace those cups of coffee with tea or, even better, green tea?

Coffee is allowed in moderation during MAINTENANCE and ATTACK. However, it's best to abstain from it during DETOX and BOOSTER. That said, if refraining from your morning cuppa creates unnecessary and counterproductive stress, then have one cup but no more.

STRESS

▶ **FACT:** Stress is fattening!

We cannot live without stress. It is essential to our survival and has been a companion both to human beings and animals since the dawn of time. So despite so many of us complaining about it, it is stress we have to thank for our survival. It's responsible for the instinctive reflex that makes us jump out of the way of a speeding motorcycle or an aggressive dog. It is also stress that turns us into supermoms (and superdads) when we need to juggle an already active life with a sick child and urgent projects to finish for yesterday. And believe it or not, it is thanks to stress that we experience great happiness when we fall in love.

This tension sends a signal to our brain to help us adapt to stressful situations in daily life. However, when it comes to health and weight management, there is a major difference between acute stress (survival instinct) and chronic stress (also called oxidative stress), as the latter has been scientifically proven to cause weight gain.

Stress interacts directly with our levels of cortisol, a hormone produced by the kidneys, which affects the way in which our body manages our energy stores (i.e., stored fat). When stressed, our body produces more cortisol, which leads to an increase in blood sugar levels.

A study conducted by Yale University in 1994 showed that highly stressed women had higher cortisol levels (logical), and that their waist fat (also called toxic fat) was greater than that of the average woman under less stress. In addition, too much cortisol can lead to a depressive state, which can, in turn, lead to overeating to combat bad feelings. Essentially, high levels of cortisol increase our attraction to sugar and bad fats (saturated fats). If you take note of what you crave when you're stressed, you will rarely notice a passion for cucumbers!

High levels of cortisol can also be blamed for increased storage of fat cells harboring toxins. Eventually, they will also affect our thyroid, the gland responsible for the metabolism of all the cells in our body, thanks to the secretion of hormones (T3 and T4). If this gland stops working properly, the body can suffer a long-term lowering of its basal metabolism (the energy we need to stay alive). If we don't compensate for this by reducing our daily calorie intake or increasing our daily activity, we will end up storing more fat.

This is why, during the DETOX phase, we shall learn how to handle chronic stress more effectively (since we cannot totally eliminate it) and, as a result, considerably reduce our cortisol and toxin levels.

A "lifestyle detox," which deals with stress as well as diet, is the key to jump-starting rapid weight loss.

HOW TO REDUCE NEGATIVE STRESS THAT FATTENS US UP

THE PROBLEM: Being Reachable 24/7

Frequently consulting our Facebook feed, answering multiple text messages, picking up all incoming phone calls, reading news throughout the day, checking work e-mails upon waking: Being constantly connected and reachable is very stressful. These interruptions mean that we don't have one true moment to ourselves. To make things worse, all these activities are completely sedentary. We become overloaded; we power through the day, relying on adrenaline, which poisons our system and causes us to pile on the pounds.

THE SOLUTION: A One-Day News and Social Media Fast

The world won't stop spinning because you don't read the news for 24 hours. You are not going to lose your Facebook friends if you don't update your status for one day. Choose, if possible, a day on the weekend so that you can take advantage of this electronic fast to go out and soak up some culture, try a new recipe, or meet with friends in person and go for a long walk in the countryside.

THE PROBLEM: Energy Vampires

Between a demanding boss who expects you to attend a meeting after work hours, when your youngest child leaves school at 3 p.m.; a neighbor who listens to loud music at the crack of dawn; the girlfriend who asks "Why do you bother dieting? You never succeed!"; and the colleague who "forgets" you are dieting and brings you cookies and sweets every single day, we are truly surrounded by what I call "energy vampires." They increase our level of stress and are responsible for some of our weight gain and our inability to lose those superfluous pounds.

THE SOLUTION: Identify and Banish Those Vampires!

Program your toxic relation's e-mails to go directly into your junk folder. Invent a serious allergy to eggs or milk in order to politely excuse yourself from eating your co-worker's cakes and cookies. Explain nicely to your boss that late meeting times can be scheduled earlier in the day. And if your neighbor listens to music at 6 a.m., suggest he/she use it for exercise and then join in for the workout!

THE PROBLEM: Poor Breathing

Being stressed means breathing poorly. And breathing poorly means bloating. The equation is very simple! How so? When we are stressed, we breathe in a shallow, or superficial way. This is because our diaphragm, which contracts and expands as we breathe, does not do its job properly anymore. Our lungs don't inflate and deflate as they should, so we take in less oxygen. A tense diaphragm causes a compressed abdomen, which can lead to intense abdominal pains and, more embarrassingly, gas. This is what gives us the dreaded and frustrating "bloated" feeling.

To appreciate how far stress affects your tummy, just think: When you are stressed, have you noticed that you sometimes need to sigh or take in an extra-large deep breath? That doing so may even cause abdominal pain? That you feel a little bloated? The big culprit here really is the shallow breathing caused by intense stress.

THE SOLUTION: Learn How to Breathe for a Flat Tummy

Discover abdominal breathing by practicing my favorite relaxation technique, "yoga breathing." This involves inflating your abdomen when you inhale through the nose (filling up deeply with air), and deflating it when you exhale through the mouth (breathing out deeply so your tummy goes flat). You don't need to force the move too much. Rather, follow your breath and let it circulate in a fluid manner. Do this for 2 to 3 minutes every time you are stressed or, better yet, when you know that stress is likely to occur. Refer to the list below for more of my favorite techniques.

THREE STRESS-BUSTING ROUTINES

PREPARING FOR A STRESSFUL SITUATION

1. Sit down with your back straight (against a wall). Imagine that you have a thread pulling you up from the top of your head.

2. Rest your left hand on your knee and shut your eyes.

3. Curl all the fingers of the right hand except your middle finger and thumb.

4. With the middle finger of your right hand close your left nostril and breathe in deeply; at the end of your inhalation close your right nostril with your thumb and release your index finger and breathe out through your left nostril.

5. Now breathe back in through your left nostril, close it gently with your right middle finger, release your right nostril, then breathe out from the right and back in again.

6. Repeat the cycle calmly for 5 to 10 minutes. Try to make the exhalation twice as long as the inhalation.

REGAINING YOUR INNER CALM

1. Lie down on your back with your eyes closed and your legs bent, feet flat on the ground, hip-width apart.

2. Breathe in on a count of 4 through your nose.

3. Hold your breath for a few seconds.

4. Breathe out on a count of 8 through your nose.

5. Repeat until you have regained your inner calm. You can take up to 16 counts to breathe out.

FIGHTING PANIC ATTACKS AND ANXIETY

1. Sit down with your back straight and your hands on your thighs.

2. Breathe in deeply and slowly through your mouth as if pronouncing the word *so*.

3. Contracting your lower abdomen, breathe out little by little, around 10 or 20 times.

4. Exhale with the sound of "hum" through your mouth. Continue for 10 to 15 minutes.

THE PROBLEM: Lack of Sleep

You know this one already: We sleep poorly when we are under pressure. Studies prove that in our fast-paced society we sleep less and less, and that this lack of sleep can be linked to:

- Greater difficulty in losing weight
- Greater tendency to pile on the pounds

Why? In simple terms: When we sleep and when our body regenerates itself we produce two hormones: leptin and ghrelin. Since leptin curbs the appetite and ghrelin stimulates it, and we produce more ghrelin and less leptin when we have less sleep, it is easy to understand how a lack of sleep can make us eat more by artificially increasing our appetite. Have you noticed that when you come back from a very late party, or after a sleepless night, you are extra hungry?

And if you think that catching up on sleep over the weekend is enough to compensate, you are dead wrong. Studies are unanimous on this: Two consecutive nights of too little sleep and the vicious circle is already in motion. In fact, a study conducted by the University of Chicago in 2012 showed that after 2 days of sleep-deprivation, participants saw their leptin levels plummet, which, in turn, increased their appetite by a whopping 45 percent! And, far from being attracted to apples, cucumbers, or raw almonds, study participants were drawn to high-energy, dense foods like pizza, salty snacks, sweets, ice cream, and so on.

Don't become too zealous: Sleeping more than your body needs won't curb your appetite, either. According to the most up-to-date consensus, you need 7 to 8 hours of quality sleep per night.

Note: Some people, like me, do not need that many hours of sleep per night. It is really a matter of finding exactly how long you need to sleep to feel fully refreshed the following morning.

THE SOLUTION: Sleep More to Lose Weight Faster

In addition to your once-weekly screen fast, replace your daily soap opera with a book and turn off the lights before 11 p.m., and you'll very quickly observe an increase in your energy levels as well as a decrease in your stress levels (2 days will suffice). Start tonight!

Consciously decide not to watch TV, stay in front of your computer, or read e-mails after 7 p.m. Turn off all lights and block out all sources of noise before going to sleep. Don't watch TV or do work in bed. Learn how to wake up to your body's natural rhythm and not to an alarm clock, which can interrupt a phase of deep sleep. During the weekend (and during the week, if you work from home) give yourself the right to take an energizing 30-minute nap (no more).

I'm sure you have plenty more tips and ideas for beating stress that apply to your own personal situation. Write them down below. By doing this, you will organize your thoughts around them and they will become a part of your normal routine.

1. ....

2. ....

3. ....

EXTERNAL POLLUTANTS

Lastly, let's talk about another source of toxins, one that is pervasive and can't always be avoided: air pollution from cars, industry, chemical products, and air conditioning.

Unless you decide to retire to the virgin jungle, it is very hard to escape ambient pollution. However, if you avoid exercising outdoors toward the end of the day, when the ozone and particle levels are at their peak, you will already be doing yourself more good in your quest for a toxin-free life. If you need to exercise when the pollution is at its peak, wear a scarf or handkerchief on your nose (as is normal practice in many Asian countries). You will be shocked to see how much soot there is on the fabric after exercising!

Switch from standard household cleaning products (loaded with chemicals) to their natural, biodegradable and environmentally friendly counterparts And if you are remodeling your house, make sure you use water-based paints and glues.

In warm weather, try to wean yourself off the air conditioning in your car by progressively increasing the temperature and getting used to not using A/C so much. In cold weather, do the opposite. This will help reduce the amount of molds you inhale (because no matter what the mechanic tells you, molds form in any system that carries air and steam).

25TH-HOUR EXERCISES

These exercises are designed to fit seamlessly into your hectic day by bringing the gym into your life, rather than the other way around. If you stand up regularly and squeeze these in, instead of staying seated at your desk for 8 hours straight, you'll notice a huge difference in your fitness and body tone. They are also great for when you're detoxing heavily—if you've started with a very toxic body, you may be more tired than usual. Aim to fit in five exercises every day.

ARM-WRESTLING

Here is an easy exercise to do at home if you have teenagers in the house or a partner who is game for it. Just ask them to challenge you to a special arm-wrestling game where your objective is not to win by touching down on the table, but rather to keep your arm in an upright position against theirs, without moving, for as long as you can. Aim to hold the position for 30 seconds, and then longer.

Do this on a daily basis. You will be impressed by the feeling of force coursing through your veins and by how toned your biceps are after a few weeks.

BATHROOM SQUATS

If you drink the right amount of water, Sobacha, and tea each day, you will find that you need to go to the restroom frequently, even if your bladder is very strong. Instead of sitting on the toilet seat, simply squat and stay in this position until you have finished. If you do this quadriceps-strengthening exercise every time you go (at least 6 times a day), you will have the thighs of an Amazonian in a few weeks, I guarantee it!

THE BRAZILIAN

You can do this exercise while brushing your teeth! We spend, on average, 6 minutes a day cleaning our teeth—that's 42 minutes per week of buttock squeezes, the equivalent of a butt-firming class at the gym, without the sweat!

1. Stand up straight, feet hip-distance apart, and bend your knees slightly.
2. Keeping your abs tight and your back straight (no arching), tilt your hips forward while contracting your glutes. Make sure you give an extra-hard squeeze as you do this!
3. Finish the move by pulling your hips back and releasing your glutes.
4. Repeat until the end of your brushing session.

HINDU PRAYER

Breasts themselves aren't muscles so we can't tone them directly. We can, however, tone what I call the "natural bra": our pectorals and an underlying muscle called the subscapularis, which is involved in lifting our breasts. I do this religiously (no pun intended) every single morning after my shower. Of course, you can decide to practice it at any point of the day—all you need is 3 minutes.

1. Stand in front of a mirror so that you can keep an eye on your posture, making sure you stay nice and straight.
2. Press your palms against each other, release, and press again, moving them upward as you do this.
3. Do a series of 20 presses above your head.
4. Slowly bring your hands down as you continue to press and release your palms against each other.
5. Repeat, moving up and down, until you reach 100 presses.

IRON BUTT

Here is a move that allows you to isolate the buttock muscles so that you can work one after the other. You can do it at your desk very discreetly; nobody will notice anything!

1. Sit on a chair. Your left leg is in a normal pose with your foot flat on the ground. Your right leg is crossed over your left, with your right ankle resting on your left knee.
2. Contract the glute muscles on the right, crossed-leg side for 30 seconds. If you feel your right side trembling a little bit, go for 50 contractions on the same side, followed by 30 seconds of deep static contraction (this is what we call isometry).
3. Repeat on the other side.

JUMPING JACKS

Do 50 of these every morning before eating breakfast, to boost your metabolism and burn calories. You can drink something first, but make sure you wait a short while before doing any jumping!

1. Stand with your legs together and arms straight down along your body.
2. As you jump, open your legs and bring your arms above your head so that your hands touch. You should land with your legs apart. Keep the knees flexed.
3. Finish the jump by returning to the starting position.

OPEN THE DOOR TO A FLAT TUMMY

Decide that each time you walk through a door, you'll suck in your abs. Once you associate the action and exercise, it'll become second nature—I contract my abs every time I walk through a doorway, without even thinking about it! Focus on contracting both your upper and lower abs (above and below your navel). You can also wear a red string or a band on your wrist that you associate with abdominal contractions, so that each time you look at it you'll be reminded to do some.

So, remember to contract your abs as often as possible, even when the phone rings, or while reading this book!

PERMANENT CONTRACTION

This is my go-to for toning the buttocks. It's easy but highly efficient. Simply contract your glutes while you wait for the bus, between train station stops on your daily commute, at the red light, in work meetings (yes, it's discreet enough!), and while cooking, washing the car, or folding laundry. You can truly do it anytime, anyplace—even while you read this book! You can choose to contract 100 times quickly or slowly, or stay contracted for one minute straight, or contract one side first and then the other. It's up to you.

WALK WHILE YOU TALK

Do you own a mobile phone (I bet the answer is yes!) or a cordless phone? How much time do you spend on the phone in a day? One hour? Two hours? More? I have calculated that I spend, on average, 2 hours on the phone every day—half of it sitting at my desk. I thus have 14 hours that I can use to walk about 6,000 steps. Put a Post-it on your phone that reads, "On the phone = walking." Just imagine how many steps you could take if you were constantly walking while talking on the phone!

If you work from home, then just walk around the block. At the office, walk around the building, in the hallways, or simply remain standing on one leg for a few seconds then switch legs and keep doing this for as long as you are on the phone. See how easy it is to squeeze in some activity? Make sure you have your pedometer on, so that you can see how many steps you have taken. Surprise yourself!

Whatever the case, always be on the move. You will burn more calories this way: 3 calories per minute for a slow-paced walk, 2 calories while standing, but only a single calorie while sitting. A whole day of regular movement can actually amount to a hefty 500 calories burned, if not more (that's the equivalent of a small burger and small fries!).

WALL PUSH-UPS

Every time you go to the bathroom, take a moment to tone your triceps.

1. Stand in front of a wall, feet hip-distance apart, close enough to touch the wall with your arms straight out, at eye level.
2. Place your palms on the wall and bend at the elbows to do 20 standing push-ups. Push your body back from the wall

harder each time, moving slowly and maintaining control. Increase the difficulty of this exercise by keeping your fingers off the wall, or by working only one arm at a time.

2-WEEK DETOX DIET

Now that we have learned about the toxins we take into our bodies through stress and external pollutants and those we generate as a result of an unbalanced diet, let's find out how we can eliminate them by means of our diet, with my 2-week program of intense detoxification. This will:

- Flush out toxins that make you feel sluggish.
- Increase your energy levels (essential for the phases that follow).
- Help you lose the first few pounds effortlessly and without depriving yourself.
- Give you back a glowing complexion.
- Establish a high level of motivation.

I ask that you follow the DETOX rules (page 23) as much as possible, as this phase is the cornerstone of my program. Just to be on the safe side, let's repeat them here. I suggest you write them by hand on a large Post-it note, which you put on the mirror of your bathroom or any other highly visible place. Writing by hand will help you better memorize the rules than if you simply copy this page or type on your computer.

- Detox your body with **5** detox foods per day. It is very important that even if you modify the menus, you stick to this magic number.
- Drink Sobacha every morning, plus 3 cups throughout the day. Sobacha is an infusion made with toasted buckwheat. The recipe is on page 69.
- Drink lemon juice with water every morning.
- Avoid red meat; cow dairy; eggs; rich sauces like tartar or hollandaise sauce; sugar products; heavy foods like mayonnaise, pizzas, or enchiladas; gluten; and alcohol, all of which can overload our system in different ways.

- We do 5 "25th-hour" exercises per day.
- We manage our stress with abdominal breathing exercises.

Just imagine you are preparing a used canvas for a new painting. Before painting over it and re-creating the new you, you need to clear away the dust, remove the old paint, and bleach the canvas (that's your DETOX phase) so that we have an amazing virgin canvas on which to draw up a healthy new life!

2 WEEKS FOR EVERYBODY?

I am often asked why the DETOX phase lasts 2 weeks, no matter how many pounds you have to lose. Simply because, in the same way that you cannot make caramelized onions in 3 minutes (you need 45 minutes for that!), you cannot cleanse your body faster than it takes to flush out the toxins. So whether you have 5 or 50 pounds to lose, the same DETOX program applies.

If your current diet is too light in fiber (fruit and vegetables), or if you are coming straight from a high-protein diet, it is very possible that these first 2 weeks will send you to the loo more often than usual. This is absolutely normal, so don't panic! It's also possible that the influx of fiber will give you a tummy ache. Add a bowl of white rice to each meal and then reduce that quantity until your bowel movements return to normal.

TOP 10 DETOX FOODS

1. BUCKWHEAT

My miracle grain! You'll see that LeBootCamp Diet recommends a roasted buckwheat infusion called Sobacha every morning and throughout the day, as it delivers so much goodness to the body. Despite its name, buckwheat bears absolutely no relation to wheat. It belongs to the same family as rhubarb and sorrel and can be traced back to Siberia, Northern China, and Japan. Buckwheat was brought to Europe during the Middle Ages by the Crusaders, who had seen "Saracen"' (as they called Middle Eastern people) using it—hence its French name, *sarrasin*. This plant is naturally organic because growing it requires no fungicides, herbicides, or pesticides—another reason why I love it. It is good for the body and good for the planet! Check out "10 Reasons to Love Buckwheat" below.

You can find bulk roasted buckwheat in natural food stores like Whole Foods, and in cardboard boxes under the name of "kasha" at very affordable retail prices in large supermarkets. You can also toast raw buckwheat groats. Just heat a large, heavy skillet over medium-high heat (do not add any oil or butter). Once the pan is hot, add groats so that they cover the bottom of the pan in a single layer. Stir the buckwheat groats constantly and shake the pan periodically to keep the groats moving. Toast the buckwheat for about 5 minutes or until the groats are browned but not burned.

10 REASONS TO LOVE BUCKWHEAT

1. It's easy to cook and has a delicious, nutty taste.

2. It's high in protein: Buckwheat contains all the essential amino acids—a rarity in nature. Combined with a source of vegetable protein like legumes, it can completely replace any source of animal protein.

3. Unlike wheat or even some types of oats, it contains no gluten, so it's recommended for people suffering from celiac disease and gluten-sensitive individuals (like me!).

4. It's high in fiber, which helps you feel fuller faster and longer, and reduces cholesterol and blood-sugar levels.

5. It has a low glycemic load—lower, in fact, than almost all cereal products. And a low glycemic load helps reduce storage of sugar in the form of fat (pp. 133–134).

6. It contains vitamins P, B_1, B_3, B_5, and B_6, all of which are excellent for our hair and skin health. These vitamins also help fight against symptoms caused by excess stress, as well as support our immune system and increase our metabolism.

7. It has a wealth of trace elements: Buckwheat contains more fluoride, copper, magnesium, manganese, phosphorus, zinc, and iron than wheat.

8. It has a higher antioxidant content than any other grain according to a study comparing the composition of buckwheat to that of wheat, oats, rye, and barley.

9. It contains several phenolic acids, which are potent antioxidants not affected by heat and transformation (i.e., cutting, puréeing, blending). Phenolic acids can help protect against certain cancers and cardiovascular diseases.

10. It has a high content of flavonoids (powerful antioxidants). Rutin, for example, has anti-inflammatory properties and can help strengthen blood vessels.

2. APPLES

Like buckwheat, the apple is a very affordable detox food. Go for seasonal organic apples to avoid those very pesticides and chemical products that we are trying to rid our bodies of! Apples are an excellent source of vitamin C. They also contain quercetin (a flavonoid and one of the numerous pigment molecules that gives color to fruits, vegetables, and medicinal plants). Quercetin is a potent flavonoid. It is used for treating conditions of the heart and blood vessels including "hardening of the arteries" (atherosclerosis), high cholesterol, heart disease, and circulation problems. It is also used to treat diabetes, cataracts, hay fever, peptic ulcer, schizophrenia, inflammation, asthma, gout, viral infections, chronic fatigue syndrome (CFS), cancer, and chronic infections of the prostate. Quercetin is also used to increase endurance and improve athletic performance.

Apples also contain pectin, a fiber that binds itself to heavy metals like mercury or lead in the colon and supports their excretion. Pectin also helps our body excrete preservatives and other food additives, including tartrazine, which has been linked to hyperactivity, migraines, and asthma. Finally, pectin is a water-soluble fiber that swells in our stomach when it comes into contact with liquids, thereby inducing a feeling of fullness. For this reason, I recommend eating an apple 20 minutes in advance of a meal at a restaurant or a buffet!

> ► **FACT:** An apple a day keeps the doctor away! The apple is so detoxifying that Russian doctors made irradiated children from Chernobyl eat apples. Indeed, many researchers, including Professor V. B. Nesterenko, of the Institute for Radioprotection "Belrad" in Belarus, established that the pectin contained in apples can help reduce radiation levels in children's bodies.

3. ARTICHOKES

Artichokes increase the production of bile. Since one of the missions of bile is to transport toxins to the intestinal tract, where they will be excreted, the more bile, the better.

Recent studies have shown that 30 minutes after the consumption of an artichoke, the production of bile increased by a whopping 100 percent. Not bad, hey?

A word of caution: Never keep a cooked artichoke to eat later. Just like broccoli or spinach, this vegetable actually releases toxins when exposed to air and light, and can thus even become toxic. How ironic when you are going through a DETOX phase!

> ► **NOTE:** Conventional guidelines recommend that cooked artichokes and broccoli can be kept for up to 3 days. Nutrition experts—such as myself— would suggest keeping them, covered and in your fridge, for no longer than 12 hours.

4. AVOCADOS

I love avocados because they are rich in healthy fats, so half an avocado (without added mayonnaise, of course) will do you good. If you add prawns and a little bit of soy sauce (but not during DETOX, as soy sauce contains gluten; instead use tamari, which has the same taste and is usually wheat free), you will have a tasty and well-balanced dish. Avocado contains glutathione. If you haven't yet heard of this, it is because the studies on this antioxidant are still very few. Glutathione enables the transformation of fat-stored toxins into water-soluble toxins, making them easier to eliminate. Also, according to a recent study conducted by Harvard Medical School in 2013, those over age 60 who consumed a lot of avocado (i.e., one a day) suffered less from arthrosis than people who did not consume avocado (with all else being equal).

5. BANANAS

Bananas are a staple food and very inexpensive. Always choose organic because the cultivation of conventional bananas is simply an ecological calamity (along with apples, bananas are one of the crops most heavily treated with chemicals). It's also a medical disaster for those living on the plantations because they are literally walking in pesticide-loaded mud. Thanks to the purchasing power of supermarkets, bananas remain very affordable, even when organic. Bananas are a fantastic source of potassium, which helps regulate the fluid levels in our body. The equation is very simple: The more fluids retained in our body, the more toxins are stored; the fewer fluids, the fewer toxins.

6. BEETS

Beets are another affordable detox food and easy to find! I prefer raw beets to cooked ones, but this is just a question of taste; both provide amazing antioxidants such as methionine and betanin. Methionine helps the body purify itself of toxic waste, and betanin helps the liver metabolize fatty acids, thus allowing it to concentrate on eliminating more dangerous toxins.

7. CRUCIFEROUS VEGETABLES

The Cruciferae family includes cabbage, Brussels sprouts, spinach, watercress, cauliflower, kale, bok choy, and other lesser-known vegetables such as romanesco broccoli, which I particularly love. Easy to find and easy to cook, cruciferous vegetables are a great gift of nature. Whether you eat them raw or not, their potent compounds neutralize nitrosamines (toxic agents produced by cigarette smoke). So, for each cigarette puff, consume one spinach salad!

Brussels sprouts also inhibit aflatoxin, a very toxic mold that has been linked to liver cancer.

With its light, peppery taste and its rich antioxidant content, watercress is a marvel of nature. It contains chlorophyll, which supports the production of red blood cells. A recent study has shown that smokers who consumed watercress daily (one salad a day) excreted more toxins in their urine than smokers who did not eat watercress (but iceberg lettuce, instead).

8. GARLIC

Garlic is a detox powerhouse and should be crushed to activate potent, beneficial enzymes such as allicin. This organosulfur helps our body maintain its pH balance (see p. 277) and can help fight cravings in smokers who are trying to quit. It binds itself to toxins such as mercury and food additives and helps the body excrete them. So don't hesitate to add crushed garlic to your salads and home-cooked meals. You can also cut a garlic head in half and roast it in the oven at 375°F for around 20 minutes—divine!

9. PRUNES

Ideal for satisfying sweet cravings, prunes contain three powerful active ingredients that work together in an amazing manner: tartaric acid and diphenyl isatin, both natural laxatives, and a type of alcohol sugar called sorbitol that can loosen the stool. Easier and more frequent bowel movements support your body's natural detoxifying functions. Plus, prunes contain a high level of vitamin C, which supports iron absorption—good news for women who are chronically iron deficient (anemic).

> ▶ **NOTE:** Eat prunes in moderation, as they contain high levels of sugar.

10. TOFU

Tofu is an amazing protein source without any saturated fat. You can replace red meat with tofu in a vegetarian chili, or you can sauté it with onions and garlic, tamari, and brown rice for an Asian dish.

Although studies on tofu's detoxifying properties are limited, they reveal that tofu binds itself to heavy metals and helps the body eliminate them. A Harvard Medical School study in 2011 showed that people who consumed tofu daily (I know, that seems like a lot!) had 10 percent fewer toxins in their body.

> ▶ **NOTE:** There has been some debate over whether the risk of breast cancer can be increased by soy products such tofu, but this is a controversial and evolving area, and the latest research showed no conclusive evidence to support this.

KEEPING TRACK OF YOUR WEIGHT

Weigh yourself on the first day of your 2-week DETOX and then at least every other day, in the morning on an empty stomach and after your first bowel movement. Record your weight on "Your Weight-Loss Progress Page" at the end of this book (page 351). Do not worry if your weight loss is not linear and constant. The body is NOT a machine and your efforts might take a few days to show results on the scale. To evaluate your progress better, I suggest that, in addition to weighing yourself, you measure your body fat (scales offering this function are becoming more and more affordable), as well as the circumference of your thighs, waist, and arms.

DETOX FOOD GUIDE

FOODS TO AVOID
- Cow dairy
- Eggs and mayonnaise
- Red meat
- Gluten
- Alcohol

Continued . . .

- Carnivorous and predatory fish (even wild fish, because of mercury)
- Non-organic fruits and vegetables

FOODS TO AVOID

- Rich sauces and heavy foods, such as tartar sauce, butter, hollandaise sauce, french fries, enchiladas, triple-cheese pizzas, and so on.
- Sugar products
- All foods containing high-fructose corn syrup
- Aspartame and other potentially unsafe chemical sweeteners (p. 30)
- Soda (whether regular or diet)
- Processed food products containing additives that may be harmful
- Processed cookies, cakes, sweets, and ready-made meals

FOODS TO ENJOY

- Sheep and goat dairy
- Non-dairy milks—almond, coconut, rice, hemp, soy, etc.
- White meat. Note that pork is NOT a white meat. This misconception is the result of a great marketing campaign in 1987 for the National Pork Board. Thanks to this marketing campaign, consumption of pork went up by 20 percent! According to the USDA, pork is a red meat. The amount of myoglobin, a protein in meat that holds oxygen in the muscle, determines the color of meat. Pork is considered a red meat because it contains more myoglobin than chicken or fish.
- Small fish (wild or organically farmed), like anchovies and sardines
- Wild large fish (salmon, halibut, etc.) from protected areas such as Alaska
- Shellfish
- Organic potatoes and sweet potatoes

- Buckwheat, gluten-free whole cereals and grains (rice, quinoa, millet, amaranth, etc.)
- Legumes
- Vegan yogurts (made from soy, almond, coconut, rice, and hemp milks)
- Mustard
- Nuts
- Olive oil, in small quantities
- Prunes and other dried fruits (organic and without sulfur dioxide), in small quantities
- Seeds
- Homemade, organic fruit juices
- Dark chocolate (70 percent cocoa solids)
- Agave syrup
- Honey
- Stevia and erythritol (natural, low-calorie sweeteners)

FOODS TO FEAST ON

- Organic fruits, especially apples, bananas, berries, citrus, and peaches
- Organic vegetables, especially artichokes, asparagus, avocados, beetroot, cruciferous vegetables, garlic, green beans, mushrooms, peas, and tomatoes
- Organic roots, especially carrots, Jerusalem artichokes, rutabagas, and turnips
- Sobacha (roasted, infused buckwheat; p. 69)
- Green, white, and herbal teas
- All spices (make sure they are not UV-treated)
- All herbs (same caution as for spices)
- Low-sugar, low-salt pickled vegetables (cabbage, carrots, cauliflower, cucumbers)
- Seaweeds
- Sprouted seeds
- Tofu

DETOX MENUS

I have created these menus with all the DETOX principles in mind: using detoxifying foods from my top 10 list (plus some other foods that have detox properties but did not make it to the top 10); avoiding gluten and red meat—but still delivering plenty of flavor. Some of my recipes can be eaten across the phases, so I have included a couple of menu suggestions from other chapters.

There's no wine allowed in DETOX, but don't worry—once you've reached the ATTACK phase, you can enjoy a daily glass of red!

The following menus are suggestions only. If you cannot follow them because you are allergic to some ingredients, or because you work long hours in an office, just pick the options that work for you. If you prefer to eat one of the dinners for lunch, this is completely fine. Repeating meals that you particularly like is also acceptable. You can also create your own options, just be sure to include at least 5 DETOX foods a day and follow all the DETOX rules.

The following tips will not only help you get the most out of your 2-week DETOX phase, but are also important principles for every phase in this book. Once you reach MAINTENANCE, they will be part of your life.

Bon appétit!

HEALTHY COOKING METHODS

The healthiest way is to enjoy fruits and veggies raw (not counting the tomato, which develops antioxidants as it is cooked). After this, cooking methods should be in this order of preference: steam briefly, grill or bake, or boil. Boiling comes last because the vast majority of nutrients are lost in the discarded cooking water.

CHOOSE ORGANIC

Remember to choose organic fish, meat, fruit, and veggies, whenever possible.

SEASON SPARINGLY

Always use sea salt—Fleur de Sel or Maldon salt are my preferences. Use it sparingly, and add freshly ground black pepper, spices, and fresh herbs whenever you like, for flavor.

REMEMBER PORTION SIZE

While the amount of fruits and vegetables you can eat are unlimited, one portion of fish or meat should never exceed 3 to 4 ounces per meal. If you have a hard time determining this without weighing, try equating the portion size to a full pack of 52 cards:

- One portion of meat or fish is equivalent to one pack
- One portion of cheese is half a pack

If you don't have a playing-card deck within reach, you can also use the palm of your hand, which is approximately the same size.

FEAST, NOT FAMINE

I'm completely against deprivation in LeBootCamp Diet. Sure, there are foods that we need to limit in all phases—particularly in DETOX and BOOSTER; but being too strict is counterproductive, as it leads to frustration and can undermine your motivation. This is why I have introduced the concept of Feast. You'll see this in the menus wherever there are fresh fruits and vegetables, which you can enjoy freely, or a super-healthy recipe where you really don't need to be strict about portion size (just remember not to increase oil or margarine quantities, if the recipe calls for them). There is always room for the occasional uplifting treat, so I've included chocolate as a snack on a few days. This will make you happy, meaning you'll produce fewer toxins! Have dark if you prefer, but milk chocolate is fine, too—again, in moderation.

DAIRY AND CALCIUM

You will notice that my menus feature hardly any dairy products. This is because during DETOX we try to avoid all cow dairy. You are, no doubt, wondering where you will get your calcium from. Despite what TV ads tell us about dairy products being an indispensable source of calcium, they are, in fact, not the only source, nor even the best one! Otherwise, how would the Japanese, who consume very little, or no dairy, survive? What's more, statistically, they have three times fewer bone fractures than the rest of the world. Remember that we are the only mammals that consume the milk from other mammals for the sake of strong bones. This has not always been the case, so how did our ancestors manage?

Suffice to say, we can get all the calcium we need from other foods such as dark leafy greens, sesame seeds, anchovies, salmon, dry figs, and some mineral waters.

DAY 1

BREAKFAST

Juice of half a lemon in 8 ounces room-temperature water

1 cup Sobacha (p. 69)

1 Sweet Buckwheat Crêpe (p. 74) with 1 tablespoon Strawberry Jam (p. 77)

1 vegan yogurt (coconut, rice, or soy milk)

■ **Feast:** Pink grapefruit

LUNCH

1 (3-oz.) tin tuna atop a salad of watercress, beets, steamed haricots verts, 1 small red potato, steamed, with Garlic Vinaigrette (p. 110)

1 Blue Boost (p. 70)

SNACK

10 raw almonds

- **Feast:** Apple

DINNER

Gratineed Scallops (p. 88)

Ratatouille Provençale (p. 103)

1 orange

DAY 2

BREAKFAST

Juice of half a lemon in 8 ounces room-temperature water

1 cup Sobacha (p. 69)

1 cup Savory Buckwheat Porridge (p. 77)

- **Feast:** Pink grapefruit

LUNCH

1 serving Pink Trout Rillette (p. 90), plus 2 tablespoons goat cheese in a gluten-free wrap

Baby spinach salad and balsamic vinaigrette with 1 tablespoon pine nuts

- **Feast:** Orange

SNACK

10 raw almonds

- **Feast:** Pears

DINNER

Steamed artichoke with Greek Cucumber Tzatziki (p. 338)

Salmon en Papillote (p. 87)

- **Feast:** Brussels Sprouts with Green Tea (p. 104)

5 prunes

DAY 3

BREAKFAST

Juice of half a lemon in 8 ounces room-temperature water

1 cup Sobacha (p. 69)

10 raw almonds

1 Hazelnut Milk Smoothie (p. 71)
- **Feast:** Pink grapefruit

LUNCH

Grilled Shrimp with Coconut Milk (p. 92) and 5 tablespoons brown rice

1 papaya

SNACK

10 raw hazelnuts or almonds

4 squares chocolate (your favorite)

1 Flat Tummy Smoothie (p. 72)

DINNER

Stir-Fried Tofu with Dijon Mustard (p. 93)

Steamed broccoli, mashed with 1 tablespoon olive oil

- **Feast:** Fresh, seasonal fruit salad

DAY 4

BREAKFAST

Juice of half a lemon in 8 ounces room-temperature water

1 cup Sobacha (p. 69)

½ cup gluten-free muesli, such as Bob's Red Mill

1 vegan yogurt (coconut milk, rice milk, or soy milk)

- **Feast:** Cubed apple with cinnamon

LUNCH

4 tablespoons Hummus (p. 111)

15 baked corn tortilla chips

- **Feast:** Citrus, Kale, and Prawn Salad (p. 84)

1 banana

SNACK

1 Sweet Buckwheat Crêpe (p. 74) with 1 tablespoon raw almond butter

- **Feast:** Seasonal berries

DINNER

Grilled Trout, Corsican Style (p. 94)

1 steamed red potato, mashed with 1 tablespoon olive oil

- **Feast:** Grapefruit-Strawberry Mix (p. 112)

DAY 5

BREAKFAST

Juice of half a lemon in 8 ounces room-temperature water

1 cup Sobacha (p. 69)

½ avocado, smashed, atop a slice of toasted gluten-free bread, sprinkled with sea salt

1 orange

LUNCH

Marinated Leeks with Herbs (p. 105) with 2 slices of ham

1 slice gluten-free bread

1 orange

SNACK

1 corn tortilla

2 tablespoons Hummus (p. 111)

5 prunes

DINNER

Garlic Scallops (p. 95)

Ginger Bok Choy (p. 106)

4 squares chocolate (your favorite)

DAY 6

BREAKFAST

Juice of half a lemon in 8 ounces room-temperature water

Sweet Buckwheat Crêpe (p. 74) with 3 tablespoons homemade apple purée (peeled, chopped apples cooked gently with a splash of water and 2 drops of vanilla extract)

- **Feast:** Pink grapefruit

LUNCH

- **Feast:** Arugula and Broccoli Soup (p. 80)

2 slices turkey breast

4 squares chocolate (your favorite)

SNACK

10 raw almonds

■ **Feast:** Nectarines

DINNER

Chicken with Lemon and Cumin (p. 96) with 5 tablespoons
   steamed brown rice

■ **Feast:** Watercress salad with Garlic Vinaigrette (p. 110)

3 slices fresh pineapple

DAY 7

BREAKFAST

Juice of half a lemon in 8 ounces room-temperature water

1 cup Sobacha (p. 69)

1 savory Buckwheat Galette with Salmon, Capers, and Dill
   (p. 76)

5 prunes

LUNCH

2 tablespoons Hummus (p. 111) spread on a gluten-free
   wrap, filled with your choice of roasted vegetables
   (peppers, zucchini, eggplant, onion, etc.)

■ **Feast:** Zucchini and Caramelized Onion Gratin (p. 107)

SNACK

5 Brazil nuts

1 small papaya

DINNER

Chicken Tortilla Soup (p. 78)

5 tablespoons steamed brown rice

■ **Feast:** Watercress salad with Garlic Vinaigrette (p. 110)

1 pear

DAY 8

BREAKFAST

Juice of half a lemon in 8 ounces room-temperature water

1 cup Sobacha (p. 69)

½ cup gluten-free oatmeal with 1 diced apple and cinnamon

LUNCH

Feta and Olive Pasta Salad (p. 85)

Sliced beets with Lemon Vinaigrette (p. 110)

■ **Feast:** Tri-Color Fruit Salad (p. 113)

SNACK

1 Sweet Buckwheat Crêpe (p. 74)

3 dried figs

DINNER

Poulet Basquaise (p. 97)

5 tablespoons brown rice

■ **Feast:** Tangerines

DAY 9

BREAKFAST

Juice of half a lemon in 8 ounces room-temperature water

1 cup Sobacha (p. 69)

1 Sweet Buckwheat Crêpe (p. 74) with 1 sliced banana and coconut flakes

Purple Milkshake (p. 72)

LUNCH

2 slices turkey breast, roasted peppers, and 2 tablespoons goat cheese in a gluten-free wrap

■ **Feast:** Pears

SNACK

10 raw almonds

■ **Feast:** Apples

DINNER

Red Snapper with Citrus and Fennel Salad (p. 98)

Steamed broccoli, mashed with 1 tablespoon olive oil

4 dried figs

DAY 10

BREAKFAST

Juice of half a lemon in 8 ounces room-temperature water

1 cup Sobacha (p. 69)

1 Sweet Buckwheat Crêpe (p. 74) with 1 tablespoon Strawberry Jam (p. 77)

1 Green Morning Boost (p. 73)

LUNCH

■ **Eating Out:** Chipotle

Salad or Burrito Bowl

Choose: Chicken or sofritas

Fajita vegetables, beans, your choice of salsa, and guacamole

(Skip the cheese and sour cream, and if you choose the Burrito Bowl, choose brown rice)

SNACK

10 raw almonds

1 banana

DINNER

Hazelnut-Crusted Trout (p. 99)

Sweet potatoes and carrots (peel and dice sweet potato, peel and slice carrots, and sprinkle with 1 tablespoon olive oil and cinnamon. Bake at 425°F for 25 to 30 minutes)

3 tablespoons Parisian Crumble (p. 114)

DAY 11

BREAKFAST

Juice of half a lemon in 8 ounces room-temperature water

1 cup Sobacha (p. 69)

1 Date Smoothie (p. 73)

LUNCH

Salmon and Avocado Roll

■ **Feast:** Oranges

SNACK

1 Sweet Buckwheat Crêpe (p. 74) with 1 tablespoon almond
or hazelnut butter

DINNER

Provencal Stuffed Zucchinis (p. 108)

French Creamy Carrot Soup (Crème de Carottes) (p. 81)

4 squares chocolate (your favorite)

DAY 12

BREAKFAST

Juice of half a lemon in 8 ounces room-temperature water

1 cup Sobacha (p. 69)

Sweet Buckwheat Crêpe (p. 74) with 3 tablespoons apple
puree (see Day 6)

1 vegan yogurt (coconut milk, rice milk, or soy milk)

■ **Feast:** Mixed berries

LUNCH

■ **Eating Out:** Japanese

Small bowl miso soup

1 salmon avocado roll (with brown rice)

1 cup steamed edamame

SNACK

10 raw almonds

1 banana

DINNER

Soup au Pistou (p. 82)

■ **Feast:** Salad of watercress, beets, and artichoke hearts in
Garlic Vinaigrette (p. 110)

4 dried figs

DAY 13

BREAKFAST
Juice of half a lemon in 8 ounces room-temperature water

1 cup Sobacha (p. 69)

1 portion Parisian Crumble (p. 114)

1 orange

LUNCH
2 slices turkey breast and ½ avocado in a gluten-free wrap

■ **Feast:** Watercress and lamb's lettuce with a vinaigrette of your choice

1 banana

SNACK
1 Raspberry Panna Cotta (p. 116)

DINNER
1 leg Chicken Tandoori (p. 100)

3 tablespoons Raita (p. 86)

5 tablespoons steamed brown rice

■ **Feast:** Green peas

1 orange

DAY 14

BREAKFAST
Juice of half a lemon in 8 ounces room-temperature water

1 cup Sobacha (p. 69)

1 buckwheat banana porridge

■ **Feast:** Seasonal berries

LUNCH
2 Parmesan-Buckwheat Crêpes (p. 75)

■ **Feast:** Salad of watercress and roasted beets with Garlic Vinaigrette (p. 110)

1 apple

SNACK

10 raw almonds

1 vegan yogurt (coconut milk, rice milk, or soy milk)

DINNER

Mariner's Mussels (Moules Marinieres) (p. 102)

■ **Feast:** Carrot-Garlic Purée (p. 85)

4 tablespoons Rhubarb and Strawberry Compote (p. 117)

DETOX RECIPES

Some of these recipes make multiple servings. You can have dinner one night and save leftovers for lunch the next day. Or better yet, share the deliciousness with your family and friends. This is NOT diet food; any food lover will enjoy these meals with flavors and textures that will tantalize the taste buds of all the foodies out there!

One more note: All of these recipes can be used in any of the phases except for some of them in the BOOSTER phase. So enjoy!

SOBACHA

This infusion (also known as soba-cha) is made from roasted buckwheat, and is widely drunk in Japan. Of all the grains, buckwheat is the richest in magnesium. Magnesium strengthens the body's capacity to resist stress, but studies show that most people don't consume enough. Here's the solution: Consume a small cup of buckwheat infusion every day and you will feel relaxed and ready to face any stressful situation!

If you can find only raw buckwheat seeds, roast them in a dry frying pan over medium heat, until golden. If you're really pressed for time, try a Sobacha tisane—such as the one I've designed for when I'm at work or traveling (see www.VOlifestyle.com).

2 tablespoons kasha (roasted buckwheat seeds)
1 cup boiling water

1. Put the buckwheat seeds in a small teapot or cup. Add the water and leave to infuse for 5 minutes.
2. Strain into another cup before drinking.

BLUE BOOST

Containing strawberries, blackberries, and blueberries, the Blue Boost brings you plenty of much-needed nutrients and phytochemicals. If you don't have a juicer, I strongly advise you to buy one! You can use a blender, then strain the juice through a very fine sieve, but it won't taste as good.

> 1 cup fresh blueberries (wild are best)
>
> 5 fresh strawberries
>
> 1 apple, chopped
>
> ½ cup blackberries (if you can't get blackberries, replace with more blueberries)

1. Rinse and pat dry the fruit.
2. Place the fruits directly into the juicer—no need to peel. Never put frozen fruits in a juicer, hence the need for fresh fruits in all recipes requiring the use of a juicer. Juice and drink right away, as antioxidants lose their potency as time passes.

HAZELNUT MILK SMOOTHIE

FOR THE HAZELNUT MILK:

1 handful raw hazelnuts

½ tablespoon vanilla extract (or less, if you prefer a less distinct vanilla taste) (optional)

1 tablespoon agave nectar, powdered stevia, or organic honey (optional)

1. The night before, soak the hazelnuts in a bowl of water. Make sure the hazelnuts are completely covered in water, as they will expand overnight.
2. In the morning, rinse and drain the hazelnuts and place in a blender, with 2 to 3 times their volume of water. Blend until the liquid turns white and milky.
3. Filter the milk through a very fine sieve or cheesecloth in order to eliminate pulp.
4. Add your choice of sweetener.

FOR THE SMOOTHIE:

1 cup hazelnut milk

1 banana

1 teaspoon vanilla extract

1 handful fresh or frozen raspberries

1 teaspoon powdered stevia

1. Mix all the ingredients in a blender and blend until smooth. Enjoy right away!

FLAT TUMMY SMOOTHIE

SERVES 1

1 cup almond milk

2 bunches fresh mint

3 ice cubes

1 pinch green tea (matcha powder)

1 to 2 teaspoons powdered stevia or 1 tablespoon agave syrup

1. Place all the ingredients in a blender and blend until smooth. Enjoy immediately!

PURPLE MILKSHAKE

SERVES 2

Serving suggestion: Can be served with an avocado sandwich for a well-balanced meal that's low in saturated fat. This makes a wonderfully fun drink for kids as well. Keep them away from processed juices!

2 cups fresh or frozen blueberries, slightly thawed, if frozen

1 vegan yogurt (almond milk, soy milk, or coconut milk)

1 teaspoon powdered stevia (or to taste)

½ teaspoon vanilla extract

2 cups plain almond milk or coconut milk

1½ cups ice

1. Place all the ingredients in the blender and blend until smooth. Serve immediately.

GREEN MORNING BOOST

SERVES 1

1 apple
1 collards leaf or handful of spinach leaves
1 celery stalk
4 strawberries
1 carrot
1 slice fresh ginger

1. Rinse and pat dry the fruits and vegetables and place them, unpeeled, directly into your juicer. Juice and drink right away, as antioxidants lose their potency as time passes.

DATE SMOOTHIE

SERVES 1

Instead of reaching for that cake or dessert, try this smoothie—it's a delicious and healthy way to satisfy sugar cravings. Dates are certainly rich but there are only four in this, so it won't make the scale tip in the wrong direction. Dates are an amazing source of potassium and fiber, while avocados are packed with much-needed vitamin E and help keep our skin supple and healthy.

1 glass vegan milk (hemp milk, rice milk, almond milk, or soy milk)
4 dates, pitted
1 tablespoon agave nectar or 1 packet Truvia
½ teaspoon vanilla extract
½ avocado

1. Place all the ingredients in your blender and pulse until fully puréed. Pour into a large glass and enjoy!

SWEET BUCKWHEAT CRÊPES

SERVES 4

This easy, gluten-free recipe is a key component of LeBootCamp Diet. You can make the batter the night before and keep it, covered, in the fridge. Serve with organic, raw honey, a tiny spoonful of low-sugar strawberry jam, or nonhydrogenated margarine. Add a piece of fruit and you have a healthy breakfast rich in prebiotics that will help you lose weight and keep you going until lunch.

⅓ cup buckwheat flour

⅓ cup gluten-free flour (my favorite is Cup4Cup; white rice flour also works well)

¼ cup water

1 cup vegan vanilla milk (my favorite is almond-coconut mix)

Pinch salt

Pinch sugar

1. Place all the ingredients in a large bowl. Whisk to form a smooth batter.
2. Heat a small frying pan over medium heat and drop in a ladle of batter. Tip the pan to spread the batter across the surface. Cook for 2 to 3 minutes. Turn the crêpe and cook the other side.
3. Set aside and keep warm while you make the next crêpe.

NOTE: I suggest you double the quantities and make more crêpes, as they freeze very well and can be reheated when you are short on time.

PARMESAN-BUCKWHEAT CRÊPES

SERVES 2

This recipe is excellent for when you are craving a savory "something." It works as comfort food without the saturated fats usually found in comfort foods. Made in 2-inch pancakes, they can be served as an appetizer with a large lamb's lettuce salad with goat cheese.

⅓ cup buckwheat flour

⅓ cup gluten-free flour

1 cup water

¼ cup aged Parmesan (see Note below)

¼ cup plain almond milk

2 pinches sea salt

1. Place all the ingredients in a large bowl and whisk to form a smooth batter.
2. Heat a small frying pan over medium-high heat and pour in a ladle of batter. Tip the pan to spread the batter across the surface. When the top is not runny anymore and the sides start lifting slightly it means it is time to flip the crêpe.
3. Flip the crêpe and cook the other side. Do a test crêpe first to determine the perfect heat level and duration for your stove. You can flip it over and over from one side to the other.
4. Set aside and keep warm while you make the next crêpe.

NOTE: Though cow's milk dairy should be avoided during DETOX, aged Parmesan is okay as its lactose has pretty much disappeared during the aging process.

BUCKWHEAT GALETTES WITH SALMON, CAPERS, AND DILL

SERVES 2

2 tablespoons salted nonhydrogenated margarine

¼ pound skinless salmon fillet

2 scallions, thinly sliced

2 ounces smoked salmon, finely chopped

2 tablespoons fresh lemon juice

1 tablespoon drained capers

1 tablespoon coarsely chopped fresh dill, plus extra sprigs, for garnish

2 Parmesan-Buckwheat Crêpes (p. 75)

1. Heat 1 tablespoon margarine in a skillet over medium heat and add salmon, cutting it into pieces with a fork as cooking progresses. When the salmon is cooked, about 5 minutes, transfer to a bowl and set aside.

2. Using the same skillet, heat 1 tablespoon margarine over medium heat. Add scallions and two-thirds of smoked salmon. Sauté 3 minutes, then add reserved cooked salmon fillet. Toss until heated through. Remove from heat; add lemon juice, capers, and chopped dill. Season with salt and pepper to taste.

3. Reheat the buckwheat crêpes in a large heated skillet, one crêpe at a time. Add one-third of the mixture onto bottom third of each crêpe. Roll up and place on plate. You can also fold the crêpe in a nice square shape.

4. Garnish with reserved smoked salmon and dill sprigs. Repeat with remaining crêpes and salmon.

SAVORY BUCKWHEAT PORRIDGE

SERVES 4

Not exactly a traditional porridge, this dish is drier, more like cooked rice. If you do like a more soupy consistency, you can add more liquid.

2 teaspoons olive oil

1 onion, finely chopped

10 ounces white button mushrooms, sliced

2 cups water or vegetable broth

1 cup toasted buckwheat

Salt and pepper, to taste

1. Heat the olive oil in a large saucepan ove medium heat. Add the onion and cook until soft. Add mushrooms and cook until soft, about 5 minutes.
2. Add water to saucepan and bring to a boil. Stir in buckwheat. Cover, reduce heat, and let simmer for 10 to 12 minutes, or until liquid is absorbed. Add salt and pepper to taste.

STRAWBERRY JAM

MAKES 1½ CUPS

1 pound strawberries (fresh or frozen), rinsed and trimmed

½ pound brown granulated sugar

3 (4 oz.) clean and sterile jars with lids

1. Place the strawberries in a large soup pot. Add the sugar and bring to a boil over high heat. Reduce heat to medium and cook for 20 to 30 minutes, stirring regularly with a wooden spoon to avoid scorching, spills, or bubbly foam on the top.
2. Fill the jars to the top while the jam is still hot and screw on the lids. Turn the jars upside down and let them cool. Store in a cool place. Best if used within 4 months.

CHICKEN TORTILLA SOUP

SERVES 6

6 tomatoes

6 tablespoons olive oil

1 teaspoon salt

Freshly ground black pepper, to taste

1 medium-size onion, roughly chopped

½ bunch celery, roughly chopped

1 fresh or dried Pasilla pepper, chopped

1 jalapeno pepper

2 tablespoons chopped garlic

4 cups chicken broth

½ teaspoon (or less, to taste) cayenne pepper

2 teaspoons ground cumin

1 teaspoon paprika

1 bay leaf

2 chicken breasts, sliced

3 corn tortillas, cut into thin strips

Juice of half a lime or lemon

2 tablespoons chopped cilantro

Diced avocado, finely diced red onion, and chopped cilantro, for garnish (optional)

1. Preheat oven to 350°F.
2. Halve the tomatoes and place them in a large bowl. Season with half the olive oil, a pinch of pepper, and 1 teaspoon of salt, and toss together until the tomatoes are well coated. Place the tomatoes on a baking sheet and roast for 25 to 30 minutes.
3. Combine the onion, celery, peppers, and garlic with the rest of the olive oil in a large saucepan and cook over medium-high heat until soft. Add the chicken broth, cayenne pepper, cumin, paprika, and bay leaf. Bring to a boil, then reduce the heat and simmer for 20 minutes.

4. When the tomatoes are fully roasted, remove from oven and peel the skins. Add the tomatoes to the saucepan along with the chicken slices, and simmer for 10 more minutes.

5. Pulse the tomato mixture with an inversion blender until smooth. Adjust seasonings to taste. Gently stir in most of the tortilla strips, saving some for garnish . Finish with lime juice and cilantro.

6. Ladle into serving bowls and garnish with avocado, red onion, reserved tortilla strips, and additional chopped cilantro, if using.

ARUGULA AND BROCCOLI SOUP

SERVES 2

1 head broccoli, chopped

1 small bunch arugula

1 tablespoon olive oil

Goat cheese or coconut cream, for serving

Salt and freshly ground black pepper, to taste

1. Bring a pot of water to a boil and add a pinch of salt.
2. Add the broccoli and arugula to the water. The water should just cover the vegetables, so add more water if needed. As soon as the broccoli is soft (about 5 minutes; you want it to be bright green) remove the pot from the heat.
3. Carefully pour the contents of the pot into a food processor and purée until smooth. Depending on the size of your food processor, you might need to purée in two batches. If you like your soup quite thick, like I do, remove some of the water and set it aside. You can always add it later to adjust the consistency.
4. Add a drizzle of olive oil, the goat cheese, and salt and pepper, to taste.

FRENCH CREAMY CARROT SOUP (CRÈME DE CAROTTES)

SERVES 6

1 tablespoon olive oil

1 onion, chopped

1½ pounds carrots, peeled and grated

4 cups water

5 tablespoons vegan sour cream

Salt and pepper, to taste

1 apple, thinly sliced, for garnish

6 fresh thyme sprigs, for garnish

1. In a large soup pot, heat the oil over moderate heat, then add onion. Heat until softened but not brown, about 5 minutes.
2. Add the carrots and cook 5 more minutes, stirring occasionally. Add water, bring to a boil, and simmer for 15 minutes.
3. Remove from heat, allow to cool for about 15 minutes, then transfer mixture to a food processor and purée. Return the purée to the pot and place over low heat. Stir in the sour cream and season with salt and pepper.
4. To serve, ladle into bowls and garnish with apple slices and thyme sprigs.

SOUP AU PISTOU

SERVES 6 TO 8

4 tablespoons olive oil

3 medium leeks, dark green parts trimmed and discarded, light green and white parts thoroughly washed and cut into ½-inch dice

6 cloves garlic, minced

2 medium carrots, peeled and cut into ½-inch dice

2 stalks celery, cut into ½-inch dice

8 cups chicken stock

Salt, to taste

1 teaspoon whole black and white peppercorns

4 small sprigs fresh thyme

4 small sprigs fresh parsley

12 green beans, trimmed and cut into ½-inch pieces

2 medium zucchini, cut into ½-inch dice

2 medium yellow summer squash, cut into ½-inch dice

1 ripe tomato, peeled, seeded, and cut into ½-inch dice

FOR THE PESTO:

6 medium cloves garlic, peeled

6 ripe tomatoes, peeled, seeded, and chopped

4 to 6 tablespoons extra-virgin olive oil

30 fresh basil leaves, washed and dried

1. In a large saucepan, heat the olive oil over medium-high heat. Add the leeks and sauté just until they start to turn translucent, about 3 minutes. Add the garlic and sauté about 1 minute more. Add the carrots and celery and continue sautéing until the vegetables deepen in color but have not yet begun to brown, 3 to 4 minutes more. Pour the stock into the pan, bring it to a boil, and reduce the heat to maintain a simmer. Sprinkle in a generous pinch of salt.

2. Make the famous Provence "bouquet garni" by placing the peppercorns, thyme, and parsley in a piece of cheesecloth and tying with kitchen string. Add to the pan. Stir in the beans, zucchini, summer squash, and tomatoes. Continue simmering until the vegetables are tender, about 60 minutes.

3. Meanwhile, make the pesto: Combine garlic and tomatoes in a blender or food processor with about 3 tablespoons of the olive oil. With the machine running, add the basil leaves, and then pour in enough extra-virgin olive oil to make a smooth, thick, but fluid paste. Transfer about two-thirds of the paste into a serving bowl to pass alongside the soup.

4. When the soup is ready, stir the remaining pesto into the saucepan, ladling some of the hot broth into the blender or processor bowl to swirl and rinse any pesto clinging inside into the pan. Remove and discard the bouquet garni. Taste the soup and adjust the seasoning if necessary.

5. Ladle the soup into individual serving bowls. Serve immediately.

CITRUS, KALE, AND PRAWN SALAD

SERVES 4

If you don't like kale because it is too tough, then think again! There are ways to make kale very tender and this recipe will prove this point!

This recipe needs to be prepared at least 8 hours before the planned time for enjoying it, or even the night before.

> 2 bunches kale
>
> 4 tablespoons olive oil
>
> Juice of 3 lemons
>
> 1 tablespoon sea salt
>
> 12 cooked prawns, chopped
>
> 2 pink grapefruits, peel and pith removed, and cut into ½-inch pieces
>
> 4 tablespoons pistachios

1. Trim the kale and remove the center stem. Use scissors to shred it in ½-inch pieces.
2. Place kale in a deep bowl and drizzle with olive oil and lemon juice. Add salt. Massage using your hands for 10 minutes. Don't hesitate to exert some pressure on the kale to "break" it and force it to absorb the oil and juice, thereby making it tender. Place bowl in fridge; every time you come near the bowl, wash your hands and massage mixture again for 1 minute.
3. After 8 hours, remove from the refrigerator and drain mixture. Place in a serving bowl and add the chopped prawns and grapefruit.
4. Sprinkle with the pistachios and enjoy!

FETA AND OLIVE PASTA SALAD

4 cups cooked gluten-free rotini or any spiral pasta, cooled

16 pitted kalamata black olives, cut in half

10 (or to taste) basil leaves, rinsed, dried, and chopped

2 cups cubed feta cheese

½ cup olive oil

2 tablespoons red wine vinegar

Salt and pepper, to taste (see Note, below)

1. Mix all ingredients in a large bowl and serve immediately. (This is not a salad that can be kept for the following day as pasta will absorb the dressing and become mushy.)

NOTE: Keep in mind this dish already gets salt from the feta cheese so make sure you taste before adding additional salt.

VARIATION: As a blue cheese lover, I have also tried this recipe with blue cheese (1 cup only) and loved it!

CARROT-GARLIC PURÉE

MAKES 1 SERVING

4 medium carrots

1 clove garlic, crushed

1 teaspoon nonhydrogenated margarine

1 pinch cumin powder

Salt and pepper, to taste

1. Boil carrots with garlic until carrots are soft. Drain and mash with margarine and cumin. Add salt and pepper.

RAITA

MAKES 2 CUPS

1 medium cucumber

1 teaspoon cumin seeds

2 cups plain, vegan yogurt

1 clove garlic, peeled and minced

2 tablespoons chopped cilantro

1 tablespoon mint leaves, chopped

Salt, to taste

Cayenne pepper or paprika, to garnish

1. Peel cucumber and grate using the large holes in your mandolin or box grater. Place in a large bowl and set aside.
2. In a small, dry pan, toast the cumin seeds over medium heat for 15 seconds until fragrant.
3. Add yogurt to cucumbers, add cumin seeds, and whisk in remaining ingredients (except garnish). Adjust seasoning if necessary. Keep in the fridge and add garnish right before serving.

SALMON EN PAPILLOTE

SERVES 4

4 (6-oz.) salmon fillets, skin on

4 pieces parchment paper

1 tablespoon fresh dill

2 medium lemons, sliced thinly

1 tablespoon capers, drained

2 tablespoons fresh lemon juice

8 pitted olives, sliced (green or black)

Salt and pepper, to taste

1. Preheat oven to 400°F.
2. Place 1 fillet of salmon on each sheet of parchment. Top each with one-quarter of the dill, lemon, capers, olives, and lemon juice. Season with salt and pepper.
3. Gather sides of parchment up over salmon to form a pouch, leaving no openings, and tie tightly with kitchen twine.
4. Place packets on a baking sheet and bake for 12 minutes.
5. Before serving, cut open the packets to release the steam.

GRATINEED SCALLOPS

SERVES 3

4 tablespoons unsalted nonhydrogenated margarine

3 small shallots, minced, divided

6 ounces button mushrooms, minced

1 tablespoon minced parsley

1 tablespoon minced tarragon, plus 6 whole leaves, to garnish (optional)

Sea salt and freshly ground black pepper, to taste

1 cup dry white wine

1 fresh or dried bay leaf

¾ cup water

6 large sea scallops

2 tablespoons gluten-free flour

⅔ cup vegan heavy cream

⅔ cup grated vegan shredded mozzarella

½ teaspoon fresh lemon juice

1. Heat 2 tablespoons margarine in a medium saucepan over medium heat. Add half the shallots and all the minced mushrooms. Cook, stirring regularly with a wooden spoon, for 30 minutes. The mixture should form a paste.

2. Add parsley, minced tarragon, salt, and pepper, and mix well. Divide mixture among three shallow gratin dishes (or if you want to make it look like you are at a restaurant, use six cleaned scallop shells).

3. Bring white wine, bay leaf, remaining shallots, salt, and ¾ cup water to a boil in another saucepan set over medium heat. The mix should slightly bubble. Add scallops; cook for about 2 minutes. Do not cook longer as the cooking will be finalized in the oven.

4. Remove scallops; place 2 in each of the gratin dishes (if using scallop shells, then put only 1 per shell).

5. Reduce the cooking liquid in the saucepan by continuing to boil it for about 10 minutes. You should see that it becomes thicker.
6. Preheat broiler.
7. To make the cream: Heat remaining margarine in a small heavy-bottomed saucepan over medium heat. Add flour and whisk continuously for 2 minutes. Add reduced cooking liquid and vegan cream; mix well and cook until thickened, about 7 minutes, mixing regularly. Add vegan cheese, salt, and pepper. Mix well. Divide the sauce over the scallops.
8. Broil until browned on top. Keep an eye on it, as the mixture quickly goes from nice brown to burned. Garnish each with a tarragon leaf.

PINK TROUT RILLETTES

SERVES 6

You'll need a ceramic terrine dish for this recipe.

FOR THE HERB VINAIGRETTE:

3 gherkins, chopped

1 onion, chopped

1 tablespoon capers

1 tablespoon fresh chopped chives

1 tablespoon fresh chopped dill

1 lemon

8 tablespoons olive oil

Salt and pepper, to taste

FOR THE TROUT:

4 cups water

¾ cup white vinegar

2 sprigs thyme

2 bay leaves

2 cloves garlic, peeled

2 teaspoons salt

½ teaspoon black pepper

1 teaspoon pink peppercorns, divided

1 fresh trout fillet (just over 1 pound)

3 tablespoons nonhydrogenated margarine

¾ cup olive oil

2 tablespoons minced chives

1 tablespoon minced fresh dill

2 smoked trout fillets

1 organic lemon

1. To make the vinaigrette: Whisk together all the ingredients in a medium bowl. Set aside or refrigerate until ready to serve trout.
2. In a stockpot, combine 4 cups of water with vinegar, thyme, bay leaves, garlic cloves, ½ teaspoon pepper, 2 teaspoons salt, and ½ teaspoon pink peppercorns. Bring to a boil.

3. Add the fresh trout fillet. Reduce the heat and simmer for 5 minutes. Remove the trout from the pot and reserve the garlic. Discard the rest of the liquid.

4. Place the trout (smoked and cooked), garlic cloves, and margarine in a food processor. Pulse while gradually adding olive oil until fully puréed. Note that due to the difference in dryness and size of trout fillet you might need a little bit more olive oil.

5. Transfer to a mixing bowl. Add chives, dill, pink peppercorns, ground black pepper, and salt. Mix well and transfer to the ceramic terrine.

6. Refrigerate covered until ready to serve. Garnish with lemon slices and serve drizzled with herb vinaigrette.

GRILLED SHRIMP WITH
COCONUT MILK

1 pound uncooked fresh wild shrimp, peeled and deveined
(see Note, below)

Salt, to taste

Juice of 4 limes

1 (13.5-oz.) can low-fat coconut milk

3 pinches curry powder

1. Preheat skillet over medium heat and spray with canola oil cooking spray.
2. When the skillet is hot, sauté the shrimp until well cooked (pink and firm when you cut a "test" shrimp).
3. Add lime juice, salt (if needed), and coconut milk. Heat briefly until coconut milk warms.
4. Sprinkle with curry and stir gently.
5. Enjoy right away, as this dish is not intended to be reheated.

NOTE: Avoid farm-raised shrimp, which contain a high level of pollutants and saturated fat because of their diet and lack of exercise.

STIR-FRIED TOFU WITH
DIJON MUSTARD

My son's favorite!

¼ pound firm tofu

1 teaspoon Dijon mustard

2 tablespoons balsamic vinegar

2 tablespoons tamari

2 tablespoons olive oil

1 clove garlic, crushed

Salt and freshly ground black pepper, to taste

1. Cube the tofu and put in a bowl. Add mustard, balsamic vinegar, tamari, and olive oil, stirring gently to coat. Add garlic, salt, and pepper.
2. Cover and place in the fridge to marinate all day, or for at least 4 hours.
3. Heat a nonstick frying pan over high heat. Sauté tofu for 10 minutes (there's no need to add any extra oil but you can add a little of the marinade to the pan, as necessary, to prevent the tofu cubes from burning).

GRILLED TROUT, CORSICAN STYLE

SERVES 3

Straight from my island, a simple yet very tasty recipe.

1 small onion, minced

7 tablespoons extra-virgin olive oil, divided

1 egg white

1 tablespoon anchovy paste (or anchoiade)

3 tablespoons chopped fresh Italian flat-leaf parsley

½ teaspoon minced fresh rosemary or ¼ teaspoon dried rosemary if fresh is not available

½ teaspoon minced fresh thyme or ¼ teaspoon dried thyme if fresh is not available

1½ cups coarse gluten-free bread crumbs

6 whole small trout, cleaned

1. To make the stuffing: Heat 3 tablespoons of olive oil in a small skillet on medium heat. Sauté onions for 10 minutes. Set aside to cool. In a separate bowl, mix the egg white, anchovy paste, 2 tablespoons parsley, rosemary, thyme, and half the bread crumbs. Add pepper to taste. Do not add salt as the fish is naturally salty and the anchovy paste does bring its share of salt. Add the onions and mix well.

2. Make 2½-inch-deep diagonal cuts on each side of fish, spacing cuts about 2 inches apart. Season fish cavity with pepper. Spoon stuffing into cavity; do not pack tightly. Close the opening using toothpicks or kitchen string.

3. To make the "panure" or bread crumb topping: Heat 2 tablespoons oil in heavy, large skillet over medium heat. Add remaining bread crumbs; sauté until golden, about 3 minutes. Mix in remaining 1 tablespoon parsley. Add pepper, to taste. Set aside.

4. Preheat a grill to medium heat. Can also be baked in oven at 375°F.

5. Brush the trout all over with remaining olive oil. Place fish on grill and cook until well done, about 30 minutes, turning after 15 minutes. Once cooked, place the fish onto a serving dish. Remove the toothpicks and sprinkle with the bread crumb topping.

GARLIC SCALLOPS

SERVES 4

1¼ pounds scallops

4 tablespoons olive oil

3 cloves garlic, minced

1 tablespoon chives, chopped

1 tablespoon parsley, chopped

1 tablespoon fresh thyme, chopped

Salt and pepper, to taste

1. In a bowl, combine the scallops, olive oil, garlic, chives, parsley, thyme, salt, and pepper. Mix well. Cover the bowl and refrigerate for an hour.
2. Heat a nonstick pan over low heat. Sear the scallops on both sides for 2 to 3 minutes per side, being careful not to overcook them. Cooking time will depend on the thickness of the scallops so always cook a test scallop first to get a better feel for it.
3. Serve right away!

CHICKEN WITH LEMON AND CUMIN

SERVES 2

This mouthwatering chicken dish has a beautiful, golden skin and a great flavor, thanks to the cumin. It's a good source of animal protein and is low in saturated fat. And even better, this recipe is easy to adapt for more people.

2 bone-in, skin-on chicken breasts

Olive oil

Sea salt and freshly ground black pepper, to taste

Ground cumin, to taste

½ lemon, thinly sliced

8 pitted olives (green or black), sliced

2 cloves garlic, thinly sliced

1. Preheat oven to 400°F. Lightly oil a baking dish and set aside.
2. Brush the chicken breasts with olive oil. Sprinkle with salt, pepper, and cumin. Transfer to prepared oven dish, skin side up.
3. Sprinkle with lemon, olives, and garlic, and bake for 30 minutes.
4. After the first 10 minutes, add 5 tablespoons of water, and do this twice more. If the chicken is looking dry, add a bit more water, but don't add too much or you'll end up with a watery sauce.
5. Serve with a green salad or steamed vegetables.

POULET BASQUAISE

A typical dish from the Basque region in the South of France.

1 (3½ to 4 pounds) whole chicken, cut into 8 pieces

Salt and freshly ground black pepper, to taste

2 tablespoons olive oil

2 red bell peppers, julienned

2 green bell peppers, julienned

1 onion, thinly sliced

1 (14.5-oz.) can plum tomatoes

½ cup white wine

½ cup chicken broth

3 sprigs Italian flat-leaf parsley, finely chopped

Brown rice, for serving

1. Season the chicken all over with salt and pepper.
2. Heat the oil in a large, heavy pot over medium-high heat. When the oil is hot, add the chicken, skin side down, and brown. Remove the chicken and set aside.
3. Add the peppers and onion to the pot, reduce the heat to medium-low, and cook for about 10 minutes. Add the tomatoes and cook 5 more minutes, then add the wine, scraping the bottom of the pan to deglaze.
4. After another 5 minutes, add the chicken broth. Return the chicken to the pot, cover, and cook on low heat for about 25 minutes.
5. Remove the chicken to a platter. Increase heat to high and reduce the sauce for 5 minutes. Season with salt and pepper, and add the parsley. Pour the sauce over the chicken, and serve with brown rice.

RED SNAPPER WITH CITRUS AND FENNEL SALAD

A typical recipe from Corsica, usually enjoyed in fishermen's villages along the coast.

4 small radishes, thinly sliced

½ bulb fennel, thinly sliced

½ red pepper, finely diced

¼ cup chopped cilantro

1 tablespoon chives

1 tablespoon finely sliced mint leaves

1 grapefruit

1 orange

2 tablespoons olive oil, plus more for brushing on fish

1 tablespoon fresh lemon juice

Salt and freshly ground black pepper, to taste

6 red snapper fillets, skin removed

1. Make the salad: Mix radishes, fennel, red pepper, cilantro, chives, and mint in a large bowl.
2. Peel the grapefruit and the orange, making sure to remove all the white pith on each.
3. Working over the bowl, cut grapefruit and orange into sections, making sure to catch all the juice in the bowl. Add 2 tablespoons olive oil and lemon juice and toss lightly. Set aside.
4. Preheat broiler.
5. Set fish on a baking sheet. Brush with olive oil and season with salt and pepper. Broil on high for 4 minutes, until fish is white throughout.
6. Transfer fish to plates and top with salad.

HAZELNUT-CRUSTED TROUT

SERVES 1

One of my first successful attempts at replacing bread crumbs when coating fish.

1 (6-oz.) trout fillet (preferably wild)

1 handful hazelnuts (or almonds, if they're easier to get)

1 teaspoon canola oil

Salt and freshly ground black pepper, to taste

Lemon, for serving

1. Place the hazelnuts on a dish towel and run a rolling pin over to reduce them into a coarse hazelnut flour. Transfer the ground hazelnuts onto a large plate.
2. Lay the trout fillet on the hazelnut flour and press to coat nicely. Turn fish over and coat remaining side with hazelnuts.
3. In a nonstick pan, heat the oil over medium heat. Cook the fillet for about 3 minutes per side, and then carefully turn over in order to keep the hazelnut crust on. Season with salt and pepper, to taste.
4. Serve the trout fillet with some lemon wedges and salad for a light meal, or with brown basmati rice for a more festive occasion.

CHICKEN TANDOORI

SERVES 2

This popular Indian dish is easy to make in your own home—you don't need to have a tandoori oven. You can remove the skin to cut back on calories and fat, if you prefer. I like to keep the skin on. This is delicious served with Raita yogurt sauce (p. 86).

¼ teaspoon cayenne pepper

¼ teaspoon paprika

½ teaspoon lemon juice

Salt, to taste

2 chicken breasts (on the bone or off) or legs

FOR THE MARINADE:

¼ cup plain unsweetened soy yogurt

¼ teaspoon cayenne pepper

¼ teaspoon paprika

½ teaspoon salt

2 teaspoons grated ginger

2 large cloves garlic, crushed

2 teaspoons lemon juice

½ teaspoons garam masala powder

1 teaspoon canola oil

Lemon wedges, for serving

Raita (p. 86), for serving (optional)

1. In a small bowl, combine cayenne, paprika, lemon juice, and salt.
2. Using a sharp knife, make three incisions on each breast. Rub the chicken with cayenne mixture. Cover and place in the fridge for 30 minutes.
3. To make the marinade, combine yogurt, cayenne, paprika, salt, ginger, garlic, lemon juice, garam masala powder, and canola oil.
4. Spread this marinade over the chicken pieces, cover, and refrigerate for 3 to 4 hours (the longer, the better—so don't fret if you find you've left the chicken in the fridge for too long!).

5. Preheat the oven to 400°F. Spray a baking dish with cooking spray.

6. Place chicken in prepared dish and bake for 20 minutes, then turn and cook another 10 minutes if using boneless chicken breast. Chicken pieces with the bone in will take a little longer. If you find that the chicken is getting dry, you can add a bit of water to the bottom of the dish.

7. Serve with lemon wedges and Raita (p. 86), if desired.

MARINER'S MUSSELS
(MOULES MARINIÈRES)

1 clove garlic, finely chopped

2 shallots, finely chopped

2 tablespoons nonhydrogenated margarine

Bouquet garni of parsley, thyme, and bay leaves

1 pound mussels, cleaned

½ cup dry white wine

½ cup vegan cream

Handful of parsley leaves, coarsely chopped

1. In a large pot, melt margarine over medium heat. Cook the garlic and shallots for 3 minutes. Add the bouquet garni to the pot.
2. When the garlic and shallots are soft, add the mussels and wine. Increase heat to high, cover, and let the mussels steam open in their own juices—about 3 to 4 minutes. Give the pan a good shake every now and then. If any mussels do not open, discard them.
3. Remove the bouquet garni from the pot, add the cream and chopped parsley, and remove from the heat.
4. Spoon into large, deep plates and serve.

RATATOUILLE PROVENÇALE

SERVES 4 TO 6

3 pounds fresh tomatoes, cut into 1-inch dice

2 pounds zucchini, unpeeled, cut into 1-inch dice

1 green bell pepper, seeds removed, minced

1 red bell pepper, seeds removed, minced

1 yellow bell pepper, seeds removed, minced

3 onions, peeled and thinly sliced

3 medium eggplants, unpeeled, cut into 1-inch dice

6 cloves garlic, thinly sliced

6 sage leaves, chopped

Basil, chopped, to taste

⅔ tablespoon olive oil

1 cup chicken broth

Salt and pepper, to taste

1. In a Dutch oven, heat olive oil over medium-low heat and sauté tomatoes for ten minutes. Remove from pot and set aside.
2. Add zucchini to pot and sauté for 10 minutes. Set aside with the tomatoes.
3. Repeat process with bell peppers, then onions, then eggplants, and then garlic, 5 minutes each.
4. Return all the cooked ingredients back to the pot, along with the chopped herbs and chicken broth, and cook on low for at least 30 minutes. If you can cook longer at very low temperature, the taste will be more intense. If the ratatouille becomes too dry, you can add more chicken broth. Adjust seasoning if necessary.
5. Can be served hot or cold.

BRUSSELS SPROUTS WITH GREEN TEA

One of my son's favorites and an antioxidant power source!

1 pound Brussels sprouts, rinsed

1½ tablespoons nonhydrogenated margarine

2 small onions, sliced

2 cups green tea, fresh-brewed (hot or cold)

Salt and freshly ground black pepper, to taste

½ teaspoon cinnamon

½ teaspoon ground cloves

1 scallion, finely chopped

1. Cut each Brussels sprout into quarters, or half if they're small.
2. In a frying pan, heat the margarine over medium heat and sear the onions until golden brown. Add the Brussels sprouts.
3. When the Brussels sprouts start caramelizing and there is no juice left in the pan, add ½ cup green tea, scraping up any browned bits from the bottom of the pan.
4. Season with salt, pepper, spices, and scallion.
5. Gradually add more tea until the Brussels sprouts are tender. If you like your Brussels sprouts on the firmer side, that's fine, too.

MARINATED LEEKS WITH HERBS

A typical Parisian dish you will find called "Poireaux Vinaigrette" on the menu of the vast majority of bistros.

8 medium leeks, white and light green parts only

4 tablespoons red wine vinegar (no balsamic here!)

3 tablespoons Dijon mustard

2 shallots, thinly sliced

8 sprigs Italian flat-leaf parsley, chopped

1 teaspoon thyme

Sea salt and pepper, to taste

8 tablespoons canola oil

1. Peel off the two outer layers of the leeks. Cut as much of the green part as to allow the leeks to fit in your steamer. Steam for 15 minutes, and set aside.
2. Prepare the vinaigrette: Mix mustard with shallots, parsley, thyme, vinegar, salt, and pepper. Slowly add canola oil.
3. Place the leeks in a plate and drizzle vinaigrette on top. Let marinate 1 hour or overnight in the refrigerator. Enjoy!

GINGER BOK CHOY

SERVES 1

2 to 3 bunches baby bok choy

1 tablespoon canola oil for sautéing

1 tablespoon tamari

2 teaspoons ground ginger (if available, 1 teaspoon fresh grated is a better option)

1. Steam the baby bok choy for 5 minutes, or according to the size of the bok choy.
2. In a large skillet, heat oil over medium heat and sauté the steamed bok choy for 5 minutes.
3. Add the tamari and ginger, and stir. Continue cooking on medium heat for 2 to 3 minutes. Serve immediately.

ZUCCHINI AND CARAMELIZED ONION GRATIN

SERVES 2

2 tablespoons olive oil

1 onion, sliced

Pinch sugar or ½ teaspoon raw organic honey

½ clove garlic, crushed

1 zucchini, sliced but not peeled

2 medium tomatoes, sliced

1 bay leaf

Thyme, salt, and pepper, to taste

1 cup chicken broth

1. Heat 1 tablespoon oil in a large pan over low heat and cook the onion until caramelized. This should take around 45 minutes, so you could use the time to contract your glutes or abs! *Do not try to speed up the process by turning the heat to HIGH as you will only succeed in burning the onions.* When the onion starts turning brown, add the sugar or honey. Remove from heat and set aside.

2. Preheat the oven to 350°F.

3. Oil an 8 x 8-inch baking dish and sprinkle with the garlic. Layer the zucchini and tomato slices, alternating to form a pattern.

4. Add the bay leaf and top with the caramelized onions.

5. Sprinkle vegetables with thyme, salt, and pepper and drizzle with the remaining 1 tablespoon olive oil. Cover with aluminium foil. Bake for 20 minutes. Remove foil and return to oven for 10 more minutes. If the gratin becomes too dry add chicken broth sparingly so as to avoid it becoming too soupy. Serve hot.

PROVENÇAL STUFFED ZUCCHINIS

SERVES 4 TO 6

This typical Provençal recipe calls for egg whites. Since we are not supposed to consume eggs during the Detox phase you might wonder why we use this ingredient in this recipe. Simply because egg whites are pure protein and are hence totally acceptable during the Detox phase.

4 to 6 zucchinis (round, if you can find them, but the classical long shape will also work)

FOR THE STUFFING:

2 cloves garlic

1½ onions

½ bunch cilantro, rinsed, plus additional, for garnish

1 pound ground turkey

1 cup whole-grain rice, cooked

2 egg whites

2 pinches cumin powder

4 pinches herbs de Provence

FOR THE STOCK:

1 tablespoon olive oil

1 cup chicken broth

Salt, pepper, and cinnamon, to taste

1 pound peas, fresh or frozen

1. Rinse and dry the zucchinis. Remove the stems. Slice a small top off each one and set aside. With a spoon, scoop out the soft center of the zucchini until you reach the end; try not to pierce through the bottom to avoid the stuffing spilling out. If you are using the classical long zucchini then cut in half and hollow out like a boat.
2. Reserve the centers in a bowl for later use.
3. Peel the garlic and onions. Chop the half onion, garlic, and cilantro.
4. In a bowl, mix the ground turkey with the chopped garlic, onion, and cilantro.

5. Add the rice, egg whites, and spices. Stir well.
6. Spoon the mixture into the hollow zucchinis and cover with their tops. If you have some mixture left, make some meatballs.
7. Chop the remaining onion.
8. Heat olive oil in a large heavy stockpot over medium heat. Sauté chopped onion until soft.
9. Place the zucchinis in the stockpot, preferably side by side. Add the chicken broth, zucchini centers, and meatballs, if you had leftover stuffing mixture. Bring to a simmer and cook until the zucchinis are fork-tender, about 30 minutes.
10. Season with salt, pepper, and cinnamon.
11. Add the peas during the last 5 minutes of cooking. Adjust seasoning if necessary. Serve with chopped cilantro, if desired.

GARLIC VINAIGRETTE

SERVES 2

1 tablespoon Dijon mustard

1 clove garlic, crushed

1 tablespoon sherry vinegar

Salt and freshly ground black pepper, to taste

3 tablespoons olive oil

1. Mix mustard, garlic, vinegar, salt, and pepper and let sit for at least 10 minutes. (If you forget it and let the mixture sit for 1 hour, it will not be a problem, as this allows the flavors to develop.)
2. Slowly add the olive oil while mixing fast with a fork.
3. Keeps 7 days in the fridge, covered.

LEMON VINAIGRETTE

SERVES 2

1 tablespoon Dijon mustard

2 tablespoons onion, finely chopped

1 tablespoon white wine vinegar

1 tablespoon lemon juice

Salt and freshly ground black pepper, to taste

3 tablespoons olive oil

1 small piece lemongrass, finely chopped (optional)

1. Whisk together the mustard, onion, vinegar, lemon juice, and salt. I don't use a blender here, as I prefer to keep the chopped onion whole. Let stand for 15 minutes minimum, but more is always better, to allow the flavors to develop.
2. Whisk in the olive oil and a few pieces of lemongrass, if using, and mix well. Season to taste with pepper and a little more salt.

HUMMUS

1 (15 oz.) can organic garbanzo beans

Juice of half a lemon

⅓ cup virgin olive oil

½ teaspoon tahini (sesame paste)

1 clove garlic

Salt, to taste

1. Place all ingredients in a food processor or blender and process into a smooth purée. Some people prefer it coarse. It is yours to choose!
2. To serve, put the mixture in a serving bowl, pour some olive oil on top, and garnish with a few olives.

   VARIATION: You can vary the taste by doing the following:
   - Add 2 teaspoons of cumin
   - Or add 2 teaspoons of paprika
   - Or no tahini (sesame paste)
   - Or add 1 cup fresh white mushrooms
   - Or be creative!

GRAPEFRUIT-STRAWBERRY MIX

1 pink grapefruit, cut in half

5 ounces strawberries, rinsed and cut in half

2 teaspoons orange flower water

1 teaspoon granulated sugar or a little agave nectar

1. Use a paring knife to slice around the circumference of the grapefruit halves and between each segment and membrane, reserving the juice.
2. Gently remove the fruit and save the peel for serving.
3. In a large bowl, toss the grapefruit sections with their juices. Add the strawberries and orange flower water and gently combine. Sprinkle with sugar, and serve in the empty grapefruit halves.

TRI-COLOR FRUIT SALAD

SERVES 3

1 pint fresh strawberries

1 pint fresh or frozen raspberries (if using frozen, thaw for at least 2 hours prior to use)

½ pint fresh or frozen blueberries (if using frozen, thaw for at least 2 hours prior to use)

Juice of 1 lemon

Stevia, to taste

Mint leaves, for garnish

1. Rinse and dry all the fresh fruit, if using.
2. Cut the strawberries in half or in quarters, depending on size, and put them in a salad bowl. Add the blueberries and mix.
3. Put half of the raspberries in a blender and purée.
4. Add puréed raspberries and whole raspberries to the fruit salad. Add lemon juice and stir gently with a spoon. Add stevia, to taste, and garnish with fresh mint leaves.

VARIATION: You can top with vanilla coconut yogurt whipped with stevia.

PARISIAN CRUMBLE

This recipe calls for berries and pineapple but you can use any other fruit you happen to have in your kitchen. The great thing about this recipe is that you can fiddle with the ingredients, the measures don't need to be precise, and the result is always delightful! If you don't have time to make the crumble mix from scratch, you can use the Among Friends brand and follow the directions.

FOR CRUMBLE MIX:

6 to 8 tablespoons nonhydrogenated margarine

1 cup gluten-free flour (Cup4Cup is my favorite)

⅓ cup buckwheat flour

⅓ cup milled flaxseed

⅔ cup almond meal

⅓ cup oat flakes

4 tablespoons brown sugar

1 tablespoon organic orange zest

½ teaspoon nutmeg

Pinch salt

FOR THE FRUIT:

6 to 8 cups fresh or frozen berries

Pineapple

3 tablespoons gluten-free flour (if using very juicy or frozen fruits)

1. Preheat the oven to 350°F.
2. In a mixing bowl, combine all crumble mix ingredients, to form little lumps (the crumble).
3. Put the fruit in an oven-safe 9 x 13-inch dish.
4. Sift the gluten-free flour over the fruit and mix it in. This will prevent the fruit from getting too wet while cooking.

5. Cover with the crumble mix.
6. Bake for 35 to 40 minutes, until crumble is browned and fruit is bubbling.
7. Let cool for 15 minutes and enjoy with a scoop of raw (coconut-based) vanilla ice cream. This dish can be kept for 5 days in the fridge (or be frozen for later enjoyment) and can be a great addition to your next brunch!

RASPBERRY PANNA COTTA

4 sheets gelatin

2 to 3 tablespoons cold water

1 cup vegan cream (soy or coconut based)

1 cup coconut milk (vanilla flavored is okay)

2 tablespoons maple syrup or coconut sugar

1 vanilla pod

FOR RASPBERRY COULIS:

8 ounces frozen raspberries

Juice of 1 lemon

2 tablespoons maple syrup

Whole raspberries, for garnish

1. Spray four ramekins with cooking spray and set aside.
2. Soak the sheets of gelatin in cold water for 15 minutes.
3. In a small saucepan, add cream, milk, 2 tablespoons of maple syrup, and vanilla pod. Bring to a simmer while stirring continuously.
4. Squeeze the water out of the gelatin and mix (with a fork) with the milk and cream mixture. Stir gently until gelatin has completely dissolved.
5. Strain the mixture into another bowl. Set aside to cool. Divide the mix equally into prepared ramekins. Put in the fridge to set for 3 hours.
6. For raspberry coulis, add raspberries, lemon juice, and 2 tablespoons of maple syrup in a saucepan. Mix and bring to a boil.
7. Remove from heat and use an immersion blender or pour into a blender or food processor to purée the mixture. Set aside to cool.
8. To serve, run a small knife around the circumference of the ramekin and carefully invert the panna cotta onto a small plate. Garnish with whole raspberries and raspberry coulis.

RHUBARB AND STRAWBERRY COMPOTE

SERVES 6

8 ounces strawberries

1½ pounds rhubarb stems

1½ ounces organic brown sugar or 5 tablespoons raw honey

½ teaspoon vanilla extract

1. Rinse the strawberries and peel the rhubarb. Cut both into pieces.
2. Combine rhubarb and sugar in a saucepan over medium heat until the rhubarb pieces are soft, then add the strawberries. Let simmer for another 10 minutes. Add vanilla. Mix and remove from heat.
3. When cool, place the compote in the refrigerator.
4. Can be served alone or with coconut yogurt.

ATTACK

GOAL:

ATTACK STUBBORN WEIGHT

AND REDUCE CELLULITE

ATTACK

> ► **FACT:** Glycemic peaks make us fat.

> ► **FACT:** Yes, we can get rid of cellulite!

RULES OF THE ATTACK PHASE

- We do one Turbo Detox (TD) Day per week.
- We drink Sobacha every morning, plus 3 additional cups throughout the day.
- We drink lemon juice with water every morning.
- We take one 30-minute walk on an empty stomach per day.
- We do one hour, minimum, of cardio per day, using the ATTACK phase to try lots of different activities. And yes, this comes on top of the 30-minute walk on an empty stomach. Try new fitness cardio activities as much as possible: Zumba, BodyPump, jogging, dancing, ice-skating, walking fast, swimming, any cardio group class, online cardio programs, DVDs, etc.
- We do two anti-cellulite exercises per day, plus as many "25th-hour" exercises as we can fit in.
- We manage our stress through abdominal breathing exercises.

Congratulations! You have completed the first hurdle—the DETOX phase—and I am rooting for you! In the past 14 days you have cleansed your body and gently slimmed down all over. As you continue to shed toxins, your entire body is starting to look less bloated, you are experiencing a new level of vitality, and, most important, you have lost your first pounds.

Your tummy is flatter; your clothes might even begin to feel a little bit looser all over. And, if you started out with a lot of weight to lose, you might already even be considering buying jeans one size down!

Let's look at your success in numbers: Check your weight first. Then measure your waist, arms, and thighs. Last, but not least, rate your energy levels. On a scale of 1 (no energy) to 10 (maximum energy), where would you say you are today?

The credit for these amazing results is absolutely all yours. So, obviously, you deserve a reward! (But not a piece of candy or a big slice of cake!) How about some new exercise gear? A pair of super-cool walking shoes? Or you might prefer a spa treatment. Hey, your body has been put through its paces and deserves to be thanked, too.

WHAT IF I CAN'T EXERCISE FOR ONE HOUR TODAY?

There are days when you will be short of time, running around, simply sick, or "the dog ate my sneakers."

It is totally okay, because we're all human! I, too, have those days when I cannot reach my ideal one hour of cardio per day. So, what to do?

1. Never, ever take a guilt trip. Guilt = stress. Stress = increased levels of cortisol. Increased levels of cortisol = increased fat storage around the abdomen area.

2. Embrace your situation and consciously accept it as not being "the end of your journey on LeBootCamp" or "the end of your diet."

3. Keep in mind that one day or even two days without the sacrosanct one hour of cardio will not derail you from your healthy path.

4. Identify your daily time thieves and see how you can arrange your schedule to carve out the time you need in the coming days.

5. Remember that you don't need one full straight hour; exercising four times a day for 15-minute intervals will do the trick, too.

6. If you have never exercised before or lead a sedentary lifestyle, it might seem daunting at first. You might even think that you will never find this magic hour. It is okay. Start with baby steps. Start with ten minutes today, twelve tomorrow, fourteen the day after, and so on. Make it happen on *your* terms.

7. Focus on the days when you were able to exercise for one hour. Congratulate yourself for this great work! Do not focus on your small mishaps because believe me, there will be a few. Only focus on your successes.

8. Without punishing yourself for not having worked out today, next time you do hit the gym or schedule a cardio routine add 15 minutes. It will make you feel better!

9. And last but not least: There is no such a thing as failing on this program. Because whatever problem you encounter, whatever hurdle life throws at you, we will find a solution and prevail!

EXTREME MOTIVATION

Is the honeymoon nearing its end? We're often happy to push ourselves for 2 weeks, but then, our motivation tends to wane and we fall off the wagon. Not here! You are not alone; I'll be right with you every step of the way.

Instead of resting on our laurels, we're now going to step it up and put new techniques in place to tackle the stubborn weight that has become part of our life and has resisted even the most arduous of diets. We are going to "Trash those pounds!" This extreme expression is actually the motto of an inspiring group of online BootCampers. I am honoring their community efforts here.

We're going to visualize those pounds removed, gone, expelled from our body; we are entering an **extreme motivation** phase. Nobody—not even yourself—will get between you and your goal. And all your weight-loss saboteurs—co-workers who bring you a 4 p.m. snack; friends who try to coax you into an extra glass of wine or the large dessert at a restaurant; the relative who gets upset if you don't have seconds—we're going to zone them all out. You're standing on solid ground and those stubborn pounds will melt, thanks to the ATTACK phase.

Our goal is to consolidate your weight lost to date and continue on this path until you have lost 75 percent of all the weight you want to drop.

MIND OVER MATTER

The mind is a powerful force when it comes to motivating yourself to lose weight. Visualization techniques help you harness this power by focusing the mind on a memorable image. Here are four of my favorites:

1. See yourself giving in: A study from Carnegie Mellon University in 2014 showed that visualizing yourself eating a meal you crave can help you avoid binging. If you're contemplating eating a specific food you know isn't the best choice, try picturing yourself pigging out and enjoying the taste of the food, which could lessen your desire or eliminate it completely.

2. Know your "enemy": When I am tired and lacking in motivation, I visualize an event in my life that is very stressful or a person whom I wish to "get rid of" (in figurative terms, of course!), and it does wonders! I know this is counterintuitive, but visualizing negative images can motivate you in two ways: either because you don't want to relive something you have already lived and did not like in the least, or they make you angry and put you in the mood that makes you want to shout, "I will show you what I am capable of!"

I guarantee that such visualizations will give you enough motivation to go on that walk, do those exercises, lift that weight, or say no to that cake!

3. Channel negative energy: For my Hollywood celebrities, I take another approach; I suggest that they think of the next casting call, of competing to get the part in their next movie. Or, if they've been left heartbroken from a relationship, I inspire them to channel their energy to get even more fit and beautiful than they were before. I call this the Vendetta Diet. Again, it's all about harnessing energy and redirecting it toward something positive.

In short, each individual should tap into his or her specific source of motivation. There's no right or wrong; the choice is yours.

4. Try new stuff: A large study has shown beyond any reasonable doubt that the participants who lost the most weight were those who were regulary trying new fitness activities. To keep you on your toes and motivated, you thus need to surprise your body with new fitness group classes (think BodyPump, Zumba, dance, stretching, or yoga), or alternate non-class activities like jogging, swimming, walking, Nordic walking, bike riding, roller-blading, etc. The more you try new ways to engage your body, the faster you will shed the extra pounds and tone your body. Avoiding boredom is key in the ATTACK phase. So, now, take a piece of paper and a pencil *(again, no computer, writing by hand will make the difference. Why? Because everything that you write becomes "reality," not easily erased like you could on a computer)* and list five new activities you will try in the coming 2 weeks at your favorite gym, and five new activities you will try outdoors. Then schedule them so that you have no excuse!

TIPS FOR PEOPLE WHO HAVE A LOT OF WEIGHT TO LOSE

On the face of it, losing weight can seem both extremely easy and daunting.

Easy, because we all know that, in principle, if we eat less and move more we will lose weight in the end. Daunting, because we know at the same time that if it were that easy we would all have perfect figures without the help of Photoshop. Daunting also because of the need for sustained motivation, of the required strength to resist the ultimately crazy and unhealthy crash diet, of the need for the certainty of our success.

I realize that losing 5 pounds before summer to look hot in our bikini is not the same as losing 100 pounds because we simply need to be in good health. The techniques we follow to shed a few pounds should never be the same as the ones we need to establish for a greater weight loss. That is why I have devised a list of ten tips specifically for those who have more than 25 pounds to lose:

1. Decide on your healthy weight and how much you need to lose to reach it. Overall and in the long run you should not lose more than 2 pounds per week, although, at first, the weight might drop off way faster than that. Divide the

Continued . . .

number of pounds you need to lose by 2 and that will give you a number of weeks in which you can safely lose your excess weight. Then, if you have followed many diets before (more than eight), add 25 percent to this number. In other words, if your result was 20 weeks, you need to add 5 more weeks to reach your goal, hence 25 weeks.

If you have more than 100 pounds to lose, you need to add another 50 percent to that total as you will need to give your body time to adjust to new weight levels along the way, benchmark, and then restart losing weight.

2. Don't be discouraged by the time you'll need to lose all the weight. Consciously accept that if it took you years to pack on the pounds, it would be unrealistic to want to lose it all in 2 months. Don't just think it, write it down and share the thoughts on social networks. It will make you feel stronger with your resolution to take the time you need, not the time your social agenda might dictate.

3. Enlist support right away. Don't put this off. Don't wait. Support for long-term significant weight loss is key. It can be your neighbor, your spouse or partner, your coach, a parent, a very, very good friend (beware of frenemies, energy vampires, or diet saboteurs), or simply a like-minded person who has the same weight-loss goal and shares the same values.

4. Establish menus for 4 weeks in advance, with healthy fast-food backup plans. Share those menus with your supporter. Carve out time to cook in advance and freeze healthy meals for the coming weeks so as to never be caught short without a right option at home.

5. Share your results on Instagram or Twitter (and you can ping me on this @valerieorsoni or #lebootcamp to get personal support from me). You can even create a specific account for this. You will be surprised by how much support you receive. Tweet your results, successes, and

failures even, and ping me @valerieorsoni for real time support as well.

6. Because after 3 to 4 weeks the dieting honeymoon usually ends, challenge yourself every week like this:

- a week without bread
- a gluten-free, dairy-free week (in addition to your TD Day)
- a meat-free week
- a vegan week
- a smoothie plus a buckwheat crêpe every morning for breakfast for a week
- 20,000 steps a day instead of 10,000 for a full week

Create your own challenges. The more fun, the better. Stimulating your creativity and constantly keeping yourself focused on new ways to challenge yourself will keep you at the top of your game.

7. Being active might not have been your cup of tea before you embarked on this journey, so you might have started in an overactive mode: gym sign-up, daily trips to the yoga studio or to the BodyPump class, etc. Now you are not feeling the same incentive to go every day, even if you are seeing results. You start to slack off. You find excuses not to go to the gym. To break this pattern, just like with the food, challenge yourself: Try one new group class per week; invite your supporter to join you in some activity twice a week and stick to your schedule; bring variety to your exercise repertoire; if the weather allows it, go swimming, biking, even roller skating!

8. Buy a new gym outfit, one size down, from a place you could not shop before. Think Lululemon, Forever 21, etc. By keeping this visible at all times in your home, your mind will get used to this new possible size for you, and it will motivate you to kick yourself in the butt and get going.

Continued . . .

9. I know you know this one but let's reinforce it: Never, ever reward yourself with food, UNLESS you cook it. Food is not a reward. Food is a pleasure that you should not deny yourself, but the price to pay is to prepare it yourself from scratch. You will be impressed at how much less we eat of the good stuff when we make it with love.

10. Be accountable, publicly and personally: Publish your blog, share it with your coach, write #noexcuse on Post-its and display them around your house. Wake up and fall asleep repeating your mantra: "Yes, I will make it happen this time."

You see, in the end, it is the accumulation of all those little steps, daily battles, weekly successes and sometimes, yes let's face it, small setbacks, that will carry you to your dream body. YOU CAN DO IT.

LET'S ATTACK!

Now let's look at some key points of the ATTACK phase in more detail. Follow these rules carefully, referring back to my hints on "extreme motivation" if you feel your spirit flagging.

ONE TURBO DETOX DAY (TD DAY) PER WEEK

You have now become an expert at detoxifying your body, so let's use this knowledge in our ATTACK phase. Starting today, you will choose one day per week for your TD Day.

You might be wondering why you need to detox again so soon after the 2-week, deep-cleansing DETOX phase. In the same way a house gets dirty with every day that passes, so, too, does your body stack toxins—from stress, lack of sleep, some fast food that sneaks in here and there—with every passing hour. Remember: Any change to your body WILL generate toxins. Even when we lose weight and exercise, our bodies produce toxins. Remain vigilant and don't let any new toxic visitors put their feet under the table!

In a nutshell: We are constantly exposed to toxins, so we need to have a cleansing schedule in place. That's where the TD Day comes in.

TURBO DETOX DAY

1. In addition to abstaining from alcohol, dairy, gluten, yeast, eggs, rich sauces, sugar products, and heavy foods (as for DETOX), stay away from all meat (you may have fish and seafood).

2. On your designated TD Day, you will consume seven detox foods. Sounds too demanding? Not at all. Check out the list of Top 10 DETOX Foods (pages 47–53).

HERE'S A SAMPLE TD DAY:

Breakfast: Freshly squeezed lemon juice in 1 cup room-temperature water, followed by Sobacha (p. 69) and Sweet Buckwheat Crêpes (p. 74).

Lunch: 1 steamed artichoke with Garlic Vinaigrette (p. 110) as part of a balanced meal of, say, grilled fish and a small salad of watercress and beets drizzled with olive oil and lemon juice, then berries. That's 5 detox foods already!

Snacks: Add an apple and a banana, and voilà!

Dinner: Choose from the DETOX menu, or create your own healthy meal—but remember to stick to the rules in point 1.

Of course, nothing prevents you from adding another TD Day when your body tells you, "I need it!"

Make sure you stick to this weekly detox day. Don't skip it. But if you forget it, don't fret because you know that if you stress, you will only release more toxins and raise your level of cortisol. If you miss a TD Day, just do it the following day.

Invite your office colleagues to follow you in this challenge. Make it a game for your little ones who can pick and choose seven foods from the list, and motivate your other half to support you by doing the same and simultaneously doing good to his/her own body.

To maximize your chances of success, choose your TD Day now and write it down in your calendar, stick a note on the fridge, and a Post-it in your bathroom. Put an alarm on your phone. This way, you simply cannot forget! And to ensure that you always have TD Day foods available, keep a complete list of them in your handbag or up on your fridge, so that you are reminded to stay stocked.

After a few weeks you will be amazed at how natural and normal TD Days have become—so much so, that not only will you not forget about them, but on the rare occasions that you skip one, you will definitely feel like something is missing!

SOBACHA EVERY MORNING, PLUS 3 CUPS THROUGHOUT THE DAY

At your first taste of Sobacha, you might have been surprised by its unique flavor, but I am sure you've gradually become accustomed to it. Do you recognize all the benefits of this millennia-old drink? It's thanks to Sobacha that your appetite is under control and you are ingesting a high level of heart-and-blood-friendly antioxidants.

I have spent long hours corresponding with Chinese and Japanese internal medicine specialists about the benefits of infused, roasted buckwheat while sipping this wonder drink. Interestingly enough when I started having a keen interest in Sobacha there were no specific studies about the benefits of my beloved beverage. Since then, though, and thanks to more and more people consuming this seed, studies are being conducted and published. A Canadian study published in the *Journal of Agriculture and Food Chemistry* showed how buckwheat can help manage diabetes, and a Danish study conducted on 857 women who consumed whole grains like buckwheat showed promising results in the levels of lignans, important cancer-fighting chemical compounds, in the blood. The world is now coming to understand how buckwheat can help us be healthier and slimmer. Stay tuned on my blog (valerieorsoni.com) for the latest studies on buckwheat.

MORNING LEMON JUICE

Now that you know that lemon juice in room-temperature water does not give you heartburn—unless you suffer from specific medical conditions—I am sure you have become addicted! And that's great news. Your skin will glow more, your energy will hit high right from the start of the day, and your liver functions will stay strongly supported.

We are going to keep the morning lemon-juice routine forever. Once again, you'll be surprised at how this has become a habit after just a few weeks. I am sure that if you miss a morning, you'll truly feel the need for it! So make sure you always have some lemons handy (organic are great, but not mandatory) and stay away from pasteurized lemon juice because the heat from the pasteurization process destroys vitamin C.

Do you feel ready? Are you mastering these three key components? I am sure that your answer is a resounding "YES!" So let's move on to another concept that is central to the ATTACK phase and to successful weight loss.

WEIGHT LOSS AND THE GLYCEMIC INDEX

Studies on using the glycemic index as a tool to lose weight were first published by the University of Toronto in 1981, based on the work of Dr. Thomas Wolever and Dr. David Jenkins, who were the first to study in great depth the impact of high-glycemic-index foods on weight gain. Numerous independent studies have now confirmed those first reports and the concept is no longer contestable. It's crucial, then, that we absorb these findings and make them part of our weight-loss journey.

HOW CAN THE GLYCEMIC INDEX HELP ME LOSE WEIGHT?

If you have ever done a glycemic test on an empty stomach you have witnessed firsthand what pure sugar does to your body. Remember that awful, very sugary drink the nurse gave you before taking blood? Remember how this made you feel nauseous? You are about to understand why!

Nutrition specialists have long categorized sugars according to their molecular structure: Simple carbohydrates (with a small, simple molecular structure) were labeled "quick sugars" and accused of provoking a blood sugar spike; the recommendation was to avoid them. Complex carbs (with a complex structure) were defined as "slow sugars" and prized for their capacity to satisfy our hunger in a sustained manner. Since the early 2000s, however, we've discovered that this classification is too simple and that simple carbs (carbs with small molecules) are not necessarily the only ones to be metabolized too fast. It seems some refined carbs with complex molecules (white rice and potato) also lead to a glycemic spike, just like pure sugar.

This discovery is what led to a new kind of classification—the Glycemic Index, which takes into account the impact on blood sugar, regardless of the molecular structure of a food, and rates foods on a scale of 1 to 100. Pure glucose has a GI of 100.

High-GI foods (with a GI close to 100) affect our blood sugar levels very rapidly. They are so quickly metabolized that they cause the body to store a lot of energy in the form of fat (glycogen). By provoking a glycemic peak, or rise in blood sugar, followed by a brutal drop, they lead to cravings and fatigue. High-GI foods include white sugar; white bread; steamed, boiled, or baked potatoes; and sweets.

Low-GI foods (with a GI close to zero) affect our blood sugar levels more slowly. They fill us up immediately and, by keeping our blood sugar low, keep us full for a long time, which means that less excess sugar is stored in the form of glycogen (fat). By preventing falls in blood sugar, low-GI foods help us fight cravings, stabilize our weight, and protect against cardiovascular diseases and diabetes. Low-GI foods include vegetables and legumes. Note that pure-fat foods like butter and oil or pure-protein foods like meat and fish have no glycemic index since they have no impact on blood sugar.

You can see why it's so important to understand the glycemic index of foods when trying to lose weight. Take my word for it—the proof will be on the scales!

Though the concept may be new to you, during the DETOX phase you've actually learned how to master your glycemic levels without even knowing it. To help you get a better understanding of what low, medium, and high GI means, I've drawn up a simple table.

GLYCEMIC INDEX	CATEGORY
<50	Low
Between 50 and 69	Medium
>70	High

WHAT IS THE DIFFERENCE BETWEEN THE GLYCEMIC INDEX AND THE GLYCEMIC LOAD?

The Glycemic Index (GI) is a measure of how quickly blood-glucose (i.e., blood-sugar) levels rise after eating a particular type of food. The effects that different foods have on blood-sugar levels vary considerably. The Glycemic Index estimates how much each gram of available carbohydrate (total carbohydrate minus fiber) in a food raises a person's blood-sugar level following consumption of the food, relative to consumption of pure glucose.

The Glycemic Load (GL), invented by researchers at Harvard University, is more precise because the GI only takes into account the sugar content of a food, while the GL takes into account the actual amount of *useable* carbohydrates, based on fiber and water content (fiber helps slow down the absorption of carbohydrates during digestion). This provides a more useful measure of the impact on our blood sugar, and hence on weight loss. That's why some foods can have a high GI but a low GL. For example, watermelon has a GI of 75 (high) but a GL of only 5 (low).

Let's have a look at the formula that calculates GL.
Glycemic Load = (Glycemic Index x number of grams of sugar in one portion)/100

GLYCEMIC LOAD	CATEGORY
<10	Low
Between 11 and 19	Medium
>20	High

Now, let's see how we can apply this formula to calculate the GL of 100g each of watermelon and white rice.

Watermelon: The GI of watermelon is 75 (high) and one portion of 100g contains 6.5g glucids. So, to calculate the GL, we multiply 75 by 6.5 and divide by 100. (75 x 6.5)/100 = 5. The answer is 5, which shows us that watermelon has a low GL.

Compare this with:

White Rice: The GI of white rice is 80 (high) and one 100g portion contains 29g glucids. So, to calculate the GL, we multiply 80 by 29 and divide by 100. (80 x 29)/100 = 23. The answer is 23, which shows us that white rice has a high GL.

Note that although watermelon is known for having a high GI, it actually has a low GL, whereas white rice is high in both categories. This means that, thanks to the research on GL, diabetics can now enjoy watermelon—a fruit that was previously forbidden. The Glycemic Load is thus a more complete indicator since it takes into account more elements than the Glycemic Index.

The GL takes into account not only the different components of a food but also the way it is cooked. Take a simple potato. When it is made into chips, its GI is 75 and its GL is 33 (both high), but when it is steamed, its GI is 65 and its GL only 14 (both medium). Why this difference? Because chips are more concentrated in glucids, due to water loss during the cooking process.

So, during the ATTACK phase, we are going to rely on GL to assess the foods we eat. This will help you lose weight quickly and efficiently because you'll understand better the impact food has on your weight. You'll be equipped with all the knowledge you need to create healthy, yummy meals that won't upset the equilibrium of your blood-sugar levels and will sustain healthy weight loss.

TRY IT YOURSELF!

1. What is the GL of a biscuit that has a GI of 75 and contains 75g of glucids for a 100g portion?
2. What is the GL of mashed potatoes that has a GI of 90 and contains 14g of glucids for a 100g portion?

Answers: Q1 = 56.25/high; Q2 = 13/medium

ATTACK GUIDE TO GI/GL OF COMMON FOODS

FOOD	GLYCEMIC INDEX (GLUCOSE = 100)	SERVING SIZE IN GRAMS UNLESS OTHERWISE NOTED	GLYCEMIC LOAD PER SERVING
ANIMAL PROTEIN			
Meat, fish, seafood	0	NA	0
Eggs	0	NA	0
DAIRY			
Butter	0	NA	0
Cheese	0	NA	0
Plain cow's milk yogurt	36	1 cup	2
Fruit yogurt	45	1 cup	5
BAKERY PRODUCTS AND BREADS			
Banana cake, made with sugar	47	60	14
Bagel, white, frozen	72	70	25
Baguette, white, plain	95	30	15
Hamburger bun	61	30	9
Rye pumpernickel bread	41	1 large slice	5
50% cracked wheat kernel bread	58	30	12
White wheat flour bread	71	30	10
Wonder bread	73	30	10
Whole-wheat bread	71	30	9
100% Whole Grain bread (Natural Ovens)	51	30	7
Buckwheat bread	72	30	8
Pita bread, white	68	30	10
Corn tortilla	52	50	12
Wheat tortilla	30	50	8
BEVERAGES			
Coca Cola	63	1 cup	16
Fanta, orange soft drink	68	1 cup	23
Apple juice, unsweetened	44	1 cup	30
Cranberry juice cocktail (Ocean Spray)	68	1 cup	24
Gatorade	78	1 cup	12
Orange juice, unsweetened	50	1 cup	12
Tomato juice, canned	38	1 cup	4

Continued . . .

FOOD	GLYCEMIC INDEX (GLUCOSE = 100)	SERVING SIZE IN GRAMS UNLESS OTHERWISE NOTED	GLYCEMIC LOAD PER SERVING
BREAKFAST CEREALS AND RELATED PRODUCTS			
All-Bran	55	30	12
Coco Pops	77	30	20
Cornflakes	93	30	23
Cream of Wheat (Nabisco)	66	250	17
Cream of Wheat, Instant (Nabisco)	74	250	22
Grapenuts	75	30	16
Muesli	66	30	16
Oatmeal	55	250	13
Instant oatmeal	83	250	30
Puffed wheat	80	30	17
Raisin Bran (Kellogg's)	61	30	12
Special K (Kellogg's)	69	30	14
GRAINS			
Pearled barley	25	1 cup	11
Sweet corn on the cob	60	150	20
Kasha	42	1 cup	10
Couscous	65	150	9
Quinoa	53	150	13
White rice	89	150	43
Quick cooking white basmati	67	150	28
Brown rice	50	150	16
Bulgur	48	150	12
COOKIES AND CRACKERS			
Graham crackers	74	25	14
Vanilla wafers	77	25	14
Shortbread	64	25	10
Rice cakes	82	25	17
FRUITS			
Avocado	10	1 average	0
Apple	38	1 average	6
Banana, ripe	62	120	16
Dates, dried	42	60	18
Grapefruit	25	120	3
Grapes	59	120	11

FOOD	GLYCEMIC INDEX (GLUCOSE = 100)	SERVING SIZE IN GRAMS UNLESS OTHERWISE NOTED	GLYCEMIC LOAD PER SERVING
Kiwi	52	1 cup	6
Mango	50	1 cup	8
Melon	60	1 cup	4
Orange	42	1 average	5
Peach	42	1 average	5
Pear	38	1 small	4
Prunes	29	60	10
Raspberries	25	1 cup	1
Raisins	64	60	28
Strawberries	24	1 cup	1
Watermelon	72	120	4
Dried fruits (figs, grapes)	65	100	38
BEANS AND NUTS			
Blackeye peas	33	150	10
Black beans	30	150	7
Chickpeas	10	150	3
Lentils	29	150	5
Cashews, salted	42	1 oz	3
Peanuts	14	1 oz	1
PASTA AND NOODLES			
Fettucini	32	180	15
Macaroni	47	180	23
Macaroni and cheese	64	180	32
Spaghetti, white	44	1 cup	21
Spaghetti, whole wheat	42	180	17
SNACK FOODS			
Corn chips, plain, salted	42	50	11
M&M's, peanut	33	30	6
Microwave popcorn, plain	55	20	6
Potato chips	51	50	12
Snickers Bar	51	60	18
VEGETABLES			
Green peas	51	80	4
Broccoli	13	1 cup	1
Green beans	30	1 cup	1

Continued . . .

FOOD	GLYCEMIC INDEX (GLUCOSE = 100)	SERVING SIZE IN GRAMS UNLESS OTHERWISE NOTED	GLYCEMIC LOAD PER SERVING
Carrots, raw	16	1 cup	2
Carrots, cooked	47	1 cup	4
Rutabaga	52	80	4
Baked russet potato	111	150	33
Boiled, steamed white potato	65	1 cup	14
Mashed potato	90	1 cup	13
Leafy greens (spinach, kale, salad)	15	1 cup	1
Instant mashed potato	87	150	17
Sweet potato	70	150	22
Yam	54	150	20
MISCELLANEOUS			
Hummus (chickpea salad dip)	6	30	0
Chicken nuggets, frozen, reheated in microwave oven 5 min.	46	100	7
Pizza, plain baked dough, served with Parmesan cheese and tomato sauce	80	100	22
Chips	90	1 cup	48
Agave nectar	30	2 tbsp	9
Honey	61	25	12

CELLULITE AND WEIGHT LOSS

Now that we have put in place the nutrition part of this ATTACK phase, it is time to tackle one major project: cellulite eradication!

Getting rid of as much cellulite as possible is an important part of our weight-loss program. What's the point in looking skinny in your bikini if your body is flabby and gelatinous? Together, we are going to take a 3-pronged approach: tackle excess weight, tone muscles, and improve the skin.

WHAT IS CELLULITE?

The official, medical definition of cellulite (also called superficial lipodystrophy, among other terms) is *"the herniation of subcutaneous fat within fibrous connective tissue that manifests topographically as skin dimpling and nodularity, often on the pelvic region (specifically the buttocks), lower limbs and abdomen."*

In simple language, cellulite is a cluster of fat cells under the skin—what I like to call "cottage-cheese skin," or "orange-peel syndrome."

WHERE CAN WE FIND CELLULITE?

You must have noticed that almost 100 percent of the time, cellulite is a female problem. Indeed, 98 percent of women suffer from cellulite compared with only 2 percent of men! This is pretty normal, since its cause is linked to the female hormone, estrogen. In women, cellulite is usually located in the lower part of the body: the hips, thighs, and abdomen.

HOW DOES CELLULITE FORM?

Cellulite can be caused by hormonal factors (water retention stemming from hyperoestrogenism that can come with menopause); genetics (blood flow, size of fat cells); and, very important, your lifestyle! Yo-yo dieting has been shown to aggravate cellulite, as does a high-stress lifestyle because it may lead to an increase in the level of catecholamines (neurotransmitters), which have been associated with the accumulation of cellulite.

But the good news is that certain dieting practices can diminish the level of these chemicals, and less body fat typically results in an improvement in the appearance of cellulite. A diet that steers clear of blood-sugar roller coasters—a low-GL diet—is ideal.

Why are we talking about the appearance of cellulite? Because a diet high in unhealthy fat and sugar leads to the storage of lipids in fat cells called adipocytes. As time goes on, the size of the adipocytes increases, which in turn leads to a thickening of the hypodermis (beneath the epidermis). The greater the lipid surplus (stored in the form of triglycerides), the more we notice a swelling of adipocytes as they fill up with fat—they can inflate up to 50 times their original size. Impressive, isn't it?

In turn, this leads to a compression of the blood and lymph flow, and an inadequate drainage of water and toxins from the body. This accumulation of waste then causes a clustering of fat cells, making the skin look uneven and bumpy—that famous orange-peel syndrome. It's a vicious cycle that you alone can stop!

HOW DO WE GET RID OF CELLULITE?

Diet: Overhaul your diet by reducing your daily intake of calories, sugar, and fat. Most important, put in place a low-glycemic-load meal plan so that your body stores less fat. In short, follow LeBootCamp Diet!

Move!: Ideally, by adopting endurance activities like walking, swimming, or bike riding. Even better, swimming in open waters will help massage your thighs and hips in ways that even a regular massage can't accomplish.

Massage: Hand massages (with the focus on tissue stimulation, lymphatic drainage, and motorized rolling techniques) or mechanical massages with contraptions like the Cellu M6 or VelaShape (available in salons) are efficient but, of course, are no substitute for a healthy lifestyle. One of the more effective ways of improving the appearance of cellulite is dry-brushing: before showering, brush your skin with a loofah in long, sweeping motions toward the heart. This will boost circulation and stimulate drainage of toxins.

Surgery and cosmetic procedures: Mesotherapy and soy-protein injections are pretty popular in France and in the United States, and have been tried by the vast majority of A-listers in Hollywood. However, some clinics carrying out these procedures use injections that have not been properly tested, and in some cases, terrible consequences, such as tissue necrosis (death of tissue), have been reported.

So, *do your homework first!* With regard to liposuction, note that while it will remove extra fat, it will not necessarily smooth out cellulite.

A lack of physical activity slows blood flow, which means it can't drain toxins efficiently. Lack of exercise also affects muscle tone, making cellulite more visible. So, a larger woman who follows a balanced diet and regular, albeit gentle, physical activity will most likely have less cellulite than a thinner woman who is inactive and follows a poor diet.

It is essential to move every day—without sweating it out for hours, but with consistency and regularity. At the end of this chapter we will review our fitness plan and look at some exercises that will help target our most problematic body zones and boost results.

ATTACK PLAN AGAINST CELLULITE

Now that we know almost everything there is to know about cellulite, let's get going and attack these unsightly lumps on our tummy, bum, thighs, and hips, in two key ways: a 30-minute walk on an empty stomach and a targeted "trouble-zone" exercise plan.

1. A 30-MINUTE WALK ON AN EMPTY STOMACH

Your primary goal is to walk a minimum of 30 minutes on an empty stomach, every morning. When I say "empty stomach," I mean empty of solids—not liquids. Before you head out, drink your lemon juice in room-temperature water, followed by your Sobacha. If you absolutely cannot walk 30 minutes on an empty stomach in the morning (it's too cold, too dark, or you live in an unsafe area; you've zero time; you're on a plane) then choose another time during the day, such as before lunch, snack, or dinner—this should be 4 hours after a meal. I am sure you can find the time!

Ideally, we should add another 30 minutes to our walking time, to reach the sacrosanct standard of 10,000 steps per day (this is the amount agreed by medical professionals across the world. I prefer to push myself and aim for 11,000). There are lots of different, free smartphone apps for measuring your steps. You build up the extra time in 15-minute chunks throughout the day, by walking to the train station or the office, and so on.

Why on an Empty Stomach?

Several medical studies (Lariboisière Hospital, Paris, in 2002; Kansas State University in 1995) have proven that you can lose weight effectively when you exercise on an empty stomach simply because you are using stored fat to expend the energy necessary to contract your muscles. These studies show that even if you burn the same calories for the same duration in both instances, when you exercise on an empty stomach you will burn 67 percent of fat, as opposed to 50 percent when you exercise on a non-empty stomach.

When exercising on an empty stomach, the body maintains stable blood-sugar levels by pumping out energy from fat stores throughout the body (from your "saddlebags," for instance). This is because the primary fat store in our liver has been used up during the night to ensure our organs are nourished properly and to maintain a stable glycemic level. This process is optimized when you perform moderate exercise on an empty stomach for a limited time.

> ▶ WARNING: The virtues of exercising on an empty stomach have been scientifically proven. However, practicing any fitness routine on an empty stomach can have adverse effects if you go beyond 30 minutes, or if you push yourself too hard by going too fast. Since your own sugar reserves are limited, if you exercise with too much intensity you will produce more toxins in your body.
>
> Indeed, if glucose is missing, our nerve cells will satisfy themselves with a replacement source of energy called ketone bodies, produced by the degradation of fatty acids (lipids). When present in large quantities, ketone bodies become toxic waste for our body, potentially leading to kidney problems or poor recuperation. We will thus avoid all problems by settling for a leisurely morning walk.

WHY WALKING IS WONDERFUL FOR WEIGHT LOSS

- Walking engages all muscle groups. While you walk, contract your abs to work your core, protect your back, and tone your abdomen.
- A regular walk will greatly improve your cardiovascular health as well as your respiratory capacity.
- Walking does not strain your joints.
- The natural balancing of your arms allows your upper body to relax and your lungs to breathe better since there is no pressure on your chest.
- Walking helps increase bone density.
- Walking burns between 200 and 320 calories per hour.
- If you have a park nearby, a morning walk is an amazing opportunity to get some fresh air in your lungs, meditate in the great outdoors, and super-charge your mind with positive thoughts.
- Walking is free and requires minimal equipment.

If the weather is not cooperating, if it is still dark, if your safety cannot be guaranteed, or if you simply don't like to walk, you can also opt to ride a stationary bike for 30 minutes, go for a 30-minute swim, or participate in any other sport that is not too intense. Choose what you like and what you will be most likely to stick to.

2. TARGETED TROUBLE-ZONE PLAN

It is proven that regular fitness activities like bike riding or elliptical cross-training, combined with strength training or swimming and dancing, will help you tone up. However, it's only through targeted toning exercises that tackle flabbiness and cellulite, zone by zone (along with a balanced diet and a regular daily walk), that you'll achieve the body you dream of—and the one you deserve.

Together we are going to get rid of untoned abs, a saggy bum, and thighs covered in cellulite. Try to do at least two or three of these exercises a day, as a minimum. To see how to perform these exercises, tune in to my blog, valerieorsoni.com, and go to the fitness section.

Let's Tone Your Tummy!

For women, a tummy that's too toned—a six- or, even, eight-pack—is not necessarily attractive, but neither is a muffin top hanging over your jeans. We are going to find the right balance by practicing easy but very efficient fitness routines *re-gu-lar-ly*. You WILL see results, but only if you lose weight at the same time: In order for your efforts to become truly visible, your body fat must be below 25 percent. (You can use a bio-impedance scale or body-fat monitor to measure your body fat. These have become quite affordable and are available online and also at some gyms.)

For your abdomen to be sexily toned, you need to target the following zones:

1. Transverse: This muscle is invisible since it is under the rectus abdominis (the one that gives you the six-pack) and serves the purpose of supporting our internal organs. This is my favorite muscle to work on as it is the easiest!

Open the Door to a Flat Tummy ▶

We first covered this 25th-hour exercise in DETOX (page 44). Simply suck in your stomach every time you go through a door. No sweating necessary and results are guaranteed!

2. Rectus abdominis: The most visible muscle.

The Plank ▶

This exercise is quick; strengthens your core (to help prevent back problems); tones your deep abs (for a flat belly), biceps, and triceps; and stabilizes your entire body. Do this exercise during the commercials when you're watching television. Use a gym mat or carpet, so as not to hurt your arms on a hard surface.

1. Lie on your stomach, resting on elbows, with hands locked together on the floor.

2. Straighten your legs and raise your body so that it is parallel to the ground. Support yourself with your elbows and the balls of your feet. Face the floor, keeping your neck and head in a straight line and contracting your abs to keep a straight back. Be mindful not to arch your back too much; this is the most common error that people make when they feel like giving up.

3. Hold the position for 15 seconds. Rest, and hold again for another 15 seconds.

    Beginners: 2 series; 1-minute, 90-second rest between series.
    Intermediate: 3 series; 60-second rest between series.
    Advanced: 4 series; 30-second rest between series.

CUT THE CRUNCH!

CONTRARY TO popular belief, abdominal muscles are among the easiest to tone and don't require a dedicated training session: 10 minutes per day is sufficient, even less if you are short on time. Above all, avoid hour-long abs or butt group classes, which too often rely on the infamous "crunch," where you push your reproductive organs down. Needless to say, this is not at all healthy for women. More and more gynecologists are screaming, "Stop the massacre!" and with good reason, because they are noticing more and more prolapses in women who have practiced too many ill-chosen ab moves. So we are getting toned—but slowly, and in the right way.

3. Obliques: These side muscles help define our waist. All side-ab exercises, or any that require a torsion of the torso, target the obliques.

The Boxer ▶

This is my all-time favorite exercise for obliques. It's very easy to do and does not require any specific equipment.

1. Stand straight, legs hip-width apart, knees slightly bent. Your back is straight and your abs are contracted.
2. Just like a boxer, you are going to cross punch: Your right fist punches out toward the left, and your left fist punches toward the right of your body. Make rapid moves and keep your hips fixed and anchored. You should not be moving your hips or legs; the move comes from your core. You will very quickly feel how your obliques are engaged in this exercise!

Beginners: 2 series; 15 punches each side, 90-second rest between series.
Intermediate: 3 series; 20 punches each side, 60-second rest between series.
Advanced: 4 series; 30 punches each side, 30-second rest between series.

TIP: Nothing prevents you (other than your neighbors, maybe) from screaming with each punch to release excess negative energy. If you are using a punching bag, you can pound to the maximum of your strength, without holding back, and you will get toned obliques even faster.

Let's Shape Your Bum!

It's very rare to hear women complain that their bum is too small! The problem is usually one of sagginess, which means our gluteal muscles need toning. Once again, I have some easy exercises to give you a sexy, firm, and peachy derrière in no time. You should already be doing 25th-hour exercises such as "Permanent Contraction" and "Iron Butt" (DETOX, pages 45 and 44) whenever you can. To sculpt your bum even further I'll now introduce you to Lunges. This killer exercise targets all three gluteal muscles:

Gluteus Maximus: If you are looking for the one muscle to blame for a saggy bum, this is it! Located behind the pelvis, it is the muscle that gives our derrière its round shape, so we will work it on a daily basis.

Gluteus Medius: This is located on the side of our pelvis. It is a very important muscle as it defines the upper part of our buttocks. It is also known as the thigh abductor because it helps stabilize the pelvis when we stand on one leg.

Gluteus Minimus: This is hidden beneath the Gluteus Medius, at hip level. It will get targeted every time you work on the other two gluteal muscles.

Lunges ▶

1. Stand straight, feet slightly apart, hands on hips. Engage your core abdominal muscles to stabilize your spine.
2. Step forward with your right foot, lifting only your left heel to allow you to advance as much as possible.
3. As you move into the lunge position, create a 45-degree angle with your right knee. Focus on a downward movement of your hips, making sure you keep your knee right above your ankle, pointing in the same direction as your toes to avoid injury.
4. During the movement, bend slightly forward at your hips, but keep your back straight.
5. To return to your initial standing position, firmly push off with the front leg, activating both your thighs and glutes.

Beginners: 3 series of 10 reps each side, 90-second rest between series.
Intermediate: 4 series of 20 reps each side, 60-second rest between series.
Advanced: 5 series of 30 reps each side, 30-second rest between series.

TIP: You can make this exercise more difficult and get better results by holding a weighted bar or dumbbells in your hands. Start with 1 pound, then 2, and advance as this becomes easy to always keep your body engaged.

Chair Bum Lift ▶

This exercise tones all the glute muscles. I do this at home (with a sturdy chair), or in the park (with a bench) when I walk my dog. You could also use the side of your bed or the sofa.

1. Lying on your back on the floor, with your bum up against the chair's front legs, put your right leg up on the seat of the chair. Grab the front legs of the chair with your hands to maintain balance and alignment.
2. Keeping your back straight, raise your left leg up to the ceiling (with foot flexed) by lifting your pelvis. You should feel a contraction right under your glutes; this is what will tone and define this area.
3. Bring your body back to the starting position and change sides.

Beginners: 3 series of 25 reps each side, 90-second rest between series.
Intermediate: 4 series of 35 reps each side, 60-second rest between series.
Advanced: 5 series of 50 reps each side, 30-second rest between series.

TIP: Breathe! Exhale when you lift your leg straight up and inhale when you bring it back down.

Let's Sculpt Your Legs!

By following my healthy weight-loss program, you are already eating well and exercising every day, so your thighs should be getting leaner as the days pass. Now we simply need to tone and define those muscles that were previously hidden under a layer of fat into gazelle-like legs!

(We won't worry about your calves as, thanks to our daily activities, they are already pretty toned and, if anything, we dream of making them smaller rather than larger.)

To tone our thighs evenly, we need to target three areas: the adductors (the inside of the thighs), the abductors (the outside of the thighs), and the quadriceps (the group of four muscles on top of the thighs). All of these exercises can be done from the comfort of your own home.

1. Adductors: Adductors are the muscles inside your thighs that help bring your legs together. They tend to sag with the years but are easy to tone if you work on them on a daily basis.

Nutcracker ▶

This is very effective for toned inner thighs.

1. Using a gym mat or towel (or on the carpet), get into a comfortable position on your right side.
2. Using your arms to support yourself, bend your left leg over your outstretched right leg, placing the left foot on the floor in front of your right leg.
3. Now raise the right leg as if you wanted to crush something between your legs. Raise the leg slowly, so that you can really feel the muscle contraction in your inner thigh.
4. Hold the contraction for a moment at the top, and then lower your leg back to the starting position.

Beginners: 3 series of 15 reps each side, 90-second rest between series.
Intermediate: 5 series of 15 reps each side, 60-second rest between series.
Advanced: 5 series of 15 reps each side, 30-second rest between series.

TIP: Add small weights to your ankles (start with 1 pound, then move up to 2 pounds, even 5 pounds) to make the movement a little more challenging and to work your muscles even harder.

2. Abductors: Abductors are the muscles on the outside of our thighs which help move our legs away from each other. When they are not toned they sag and are often called "saddlebags." They visually add 10 pounds to a body. Hence, it is very important to work on our abductors daily.

Gazelle Legs ▶

This is great for getting rid of saddlebags.

1. Using a gym mat, towel, or the carpet, find a comfortable position on your right side. Keep your core strong and don't arch your back.
2. Using your arms to support yourself, keep your upper body upright and very gently raise your left leg in a controlled movement. Keep your foot pointed like a dancer, or flex it to work your muscles differently.
3. Lower your leg gently, always remaining in control of the movement.

> **TIP:** Close your eyes when you do this exercise so that you can focus on feeling the muscle work and establish the muscle-brain connection, to engage muscles more fully. You can also do this movement in front of a mirror to make sure your position is perfect.

> **Beginners:** 3 series of 25 reps each side, 90-second rest between series.
> **Intermediate:** 4 series of 35 reps each side, 60-second rest between series.
> **Advanced:** 5 series of 50 reps each side with 1-pound ankle weights, then move up to 2 pounds, even 4 pounds, 30-second rest between series.

3. Quadriceps: This group of four muscles at the top of the thighs is even easier to tone than the adductors and abductors. But you know this, as you should already be doing my 25th-hour exercise: "Bathroom Squats" (DETOX, page 42). Here's another 25th-hour exercise—it's my favorite for toning the thighs.

Invisible Chair ▶

Do this 25th-hour exercise while waiting for the kettle to boil, in the elevator, or with a Swiss Ball against the wall.

1. Lean your back flat against a wall with your feet shoulder-width apart. Your heels should be 10 to 15 inches from the wall.

2. Slide down the wall until you look as if you're sitting on a chair. Your legs should be at a 90-degree angle. Make sure your back is flat and your knees don't go over your toes; otherwise, you may create unnecessary pressure in your knee joints.

3. Hold for as long as you can (from 30 seconds to 2 minutes, or until the kettle boils or the elevator doors open). Then rest and repeat.

BE STRONG!

I strongly suggest you do not move on to the last phase (MAINTENANCE) until you have shed 75 percent of the weight you want to lose.

For instance, if you started with 11 pounds to lose, you can progress to the next phase once you have lost 8 pounds. And if you started with 44 pounds to lose, don't proceed to MAINTENANCE until you have lost 37 pounds.

I know how frustrating it can be not to shed more than a couple of pounds per week when you have a lot to lose, especially if you are surrounded by friends who lose weight rapidly on dangerous and depriving diets. But remember that they have a problem—a big one! An unbalanced diet with lots of deprivation means a body that will avenge itself the very instant you take the slightest detour from the prescribed regimen.

Keep in mind that everyone's rate of weight loss is different. Some people can lose a couple of pounds a week, while others lose more slowly. Don't despair. Consistent weight loss of 2 pounds a week is a myth that causes us to get frustrated and sabotage our efforts. A host of factors (more sodium, hormonal fluctuations, etc.) can affect how much weight we lose each week. You just want to aim for a trend of steady weight loss. And after the DETOX stage, where you might lose more quickly (due to loss of water or if you have a lot to lose), you never want to lose more than 2 pounds per week. True, if your starting point is extremely high and if your diet has been poor for years, it is totally possible that you will lose more than 2 pounds per week. I have had BootCampers who started their journey with me with more than 100 pounds to lose. During their first few weeks they did lose an average of 3 to 4 pounds a week and this is totally fine. However, for those who do not need to shed more than 20 pounds, it is important to keep the weight loss steady and slow enough for your body to acquire your new YOU. If you feel you are losing too quickly I am begging you to not stay in this fast lane and instead go into bench-marking mode (see page 157) to benchmark your weight and establish a new set point. This is the only way for you to lose and never regain, which is what my program is about.

So, BE STRONG. I am here all the way with you.

TOP 10 WEIGHT-LOSS TIPS

1. I BUY FOODS I DON'T "LIKE"

If you are, like me, a seriously insatiable gourmand—in other words, you cannot resist the temptations your house harbors—you need an infallible strategy so that you never fall prey to those traps that lurk in the cupboards.

My solution? When it comes to treats, I choose flavors I don't like when I shop (or bake) for my family. Ice cream? Orange sher-bert, the only ice cream flavor I don't care for—but, luckily, my family loves! Cake? Coffee. I really don't like the taste of coffee.

You know by now that I am a true advocate of delicious food and would never miss an occasion to thrill my taste buds. But, I want to do so on my terms, not by falling into hidden traps.

And you? Which tastes and flavors don't you like? From now on, these will guide how you shop. Of course, this works only if your tastes are different from those of your family. If they aren't . . . don't buy treats in the first place!

2. I BLOG

To make sure I stay on the right path I keep a blog—a public one (valerieorsoni.com) and a private, little one, where I jot down my weight, body fat, thigh circumference, waist, and so on. I encourage you to take your measurements regularly—you will be so pleased to see your results that this will make you happy!

I am frequently asked, "How often should I weigh myself?" There is no perfect rule but, apart from during DETOX where I suggest a daily weigh-in, I recommend you weigh yourself every week.

However, some people prefer to keep a tight rein on their weight. For them (and me), a daily morning weigh-in becomes part of our routine, just like brushing your teeth or taking a shower. As long as this does not become an obsession, you are fine.

3. I CREATE A WEIGHT-LOSS PHOTO ALBUM

Take pictures of yourself! This will do wonders if you have a lot of weight to lose. To make this experience as positive as possible, I suggest you take a picture each week, in the same place, in the same outfit. At the end of your journey you will be able to create a surprising slideshow of your figure's evolution with time.

Make sure you take pictures of yourself from different angles (profile, face, back; zooming in on certain trouble zones) so as to fully appreciate your fantastic results down the line.

4. I EXERCISE EFFORTLESSLY THANKS TO MY "25TH-HOUR" EXERCISES (SEE DETOX, PAGE 42)

5. I USE MINT TO SUPPRESS MY APPETITE

This tip is totally empirical and stems from my personal experience, which I have shared with numerous BootCampers over the years. Chew mint-flavored gum at the end of the meal, or brush your teeth with a mint toothpaste. You'll be amazed at how you are no longer attracted to that piece of cheesecake or big brownie.

When you need to attend a party or function with a tempting buffet, arrive (discreetly) chewing mint gum so that you spend your first few minutes doing this instead of jumping on the rich foods. Empirical studies have shown that this tip can help you curb your appetite by 25 percent. Don't forget to choose a chewing gum that does not contain toxic sweeteners (see page 29).

Continued . . .

6. I BUY MYSELF A NICE PIECE OF JEWELRY WHEN I'M SUCCESSFUL AT LOSING WEIGHT

Do you love jewels? If the answer is yes, then give yourself a bracelet, a pendant, a necklace, a ring, or even a nice ribbon to tie around your wrist. It doesn't have to be expensive—it could come from a thrift shop, a store like Forever 21, or be home-made. This will remind you of your weight-loss goals throughout the day.

If you need an extra prompt, choose a bracelet with charms that make a noise when you move. This noise will guarantee you keep your eyes on the prize: namely, your dream body!

7. I AIM FOR ONE NOTCH DOWN ON MY BELT

Write on the inside of your belt, "I want to get to this notch," with a little arrow. Of course, nobody will see this motivational state-ment but you. Make sure you do this for the next notch and the one after that . . . until you have reached your dream waist size.

8. TEA SIGNALS THE END OF THE MEAL

If, like me, you like to end a meal on a sweet note, a square of chocolate or two spoonfuls of your companion's dessert (my fa-vorite solution!) does the trick.

The problem is that we very rarely stop after those two spoon-fuls because we are also tempted to finish the whole plate, to polish off our kids' desserts, and so on. Without realizing it, we end up eating more than 200 calories. Remember that to produce one pound of fat you need 3,500 excess calories; so at a rate of 200 calories per day, that would take only 17 days. Scary, isn't it?

A nice cup of tea is my absolute signal that the meal is over. And to help keep a flat tummy I usually go for an infusion of fresh mint (with no black or green tea added, and no milk), which reduces bloating.

9. I LEAVE MY PHOTO ON THE FRIDGE

I often read in women's magazines that nothing beats the picture of a very overweight lady taped on the fridge door, to prevent you from opening it and gorging yourself. I have a radically op-posite approach: If you constantly see an overweight person (you or somebody else) you'll soon begin thinking this is the new norm.

That's why I prefer to do the reverse: Find a picture of yourself when you had your dream body, or choose a celeb whose body looks healthy and simply amazing. Then glue a cutout of your face on top of her body and place this picture on your fridge. Each time you lay eyes on this picture you will subconsciously think, "I want to look hot, too. I can do it!" or, "How about I go for a 30-minute walk?"

IMPORTANT NOTE: *Please* don't go for an unhealthy, skinny girl, okay? Your goal should be, first and foremost, to be the healthiest that you can be—I'm not suggesting you try and turn into someone else!

10. I NEVER, EVER WAIT FOR THE ELEVATOR

The University of South Carolina–Aiken has conducted an interesting study that concludes that since elevators always take some time to arrive, if you take the stairs instead you will gain an average of 20 seconds. (In this study, the stairs were within view of the elevator.)

This amusing finding points to one conclusion: Save time, tone your thighs, mold your calves, and slim your ankles by taking the stairs. Those "gazelle legs" are within your reach!

PLATEAUS AND BENCHMARKING

As I told you in the introduction, I had weight issues of my own in a faraway past (well, not that far away!). Diet after diet, there was always that one thing that drove me crazy: the dreaded "plateau." I'm sure you have found the same.

You have been at it for weeks, sweating at the gym, rationing yourself and depriving yourself of a social life, but you've got to a point where the scales show no sign of tipping in the right direction. Argh! So, what the heck? You might as well have that giant, steaming pizza or the whole tub of ice cream. You're massively frustrated, and you'll get your revenge. Won't you?

This all happens for a reason: You have been tricked into believing that your weight will drop steadily should you follow the program to the letter. When you realized your hard work was not paying off, you might have gone online and consulted blogs and forums, only to be told that you're not following the diet properly. Infuriating! And likely to have you wracking your brain to work out where you went wrong.

So why all this confusion? Because on top of being taunted by images of successful dieters, the message distilled to you is: "You *will* lose two pounds a week." You have been led to believe that weight loss is a steady curve. You are under the false impression that you HAVE to lose some every week or else you are plateauing—and this is not acceptable.

Well, let me tell you something: You have been deceived! My numerous years of coaching thousands of women of all ages and sizes have led me to embrace plateaus. In fact, I welcome them. I ask for them, even. I have discovered what they are really about and how they form new points of reference for us to use. This is what I call "benchmarking."

WHAT IS A PLATEAU?

A plateau defines the moment in a weight-loss journey where the dieter stops losing weight even though she or he is still following a healthy diet and fitness regimen.

WHY DOES A PLATEAU OCCUR?

Here's how it works:

- You reduce your caloric intake. Since your body needs energy to function, it releases its stores of glycogen (fat contained in the liver and in the muscles). Because glycogen binds to water, when it gets burned by the body for energy it releases a large amount of water. This leads to a rapid weight drop.
- You feel happy about this and you might not watch your diet as well as when you started out. You might even scale down a little on your physical activity.
- Because your overall muscle mass has dropped (remember, glycogen is stored in the muscles), your metabolism slows down.
- Because you eat less, your metabolism slows down even more to conserve more energy.

At that point you burn exactly what you eat and you have hit a plateau.

Some people—very few—never hit a plateau. For them, weight loss is linear. They are an exception to the rule. However, the average dieter will experience plateaus.

My willingness to embrace plateaus led to my theory of "benchmarking," which has since been proven to be effective by BootCampers.

WHAT DOES BENCHMARKING MEAN?

The original meaning of benchmark is, "A measure used to judge the level of something." But now I'm going to take this definition and apply it to weight loss.

We're going to take your plateau weight and use it as a benchmark, or reference point. Then, we're going to work on this plateau weight to trick your mind into thinking this is your new, heaviest weight ever.

To achieve this state of mind requires some work on your part. Decide consciously that, if it took you years to gain 20 pounds, or even 100 pounds, or more, it makes sense that your body needs time to readjust to a lighter self as you shed the pounds.

Embrace your plateau by thinking, "If my body is not shedding weight now, it is because it needs time to adjust to the new ME." In truth, your body and your mind will resist change. But we all know that change is welcome when it comes to our health, well-being, and happiness. Several blood tests have shown that when a dieter reaches a plateau her body is working hard at rebalancing certain elements that have been impacted adversely by the weight loss, even when following a healthy weight-loss plan.

Remind yourself that your body is not a machine, but a gracious, elegant, and very delicate organism, which might not respond to having its buttons pushed as if it were a robot. As you lose weight, hormonal levels can change, as will most certainly potassium levels and in general, fluid levels. They need to adjust in order to find their new equilibrium. When we thought our body was resisting change it was in fact working hard at finding its perfect state of balance where all body functions are at their optimum.

This is one of the reasons why your weight loss doesn't always follow a straight line.

HOW LONG SHOULD A
PLATEAU LAST?

Based on my empirical experience, each plateau should last, in weeks, one-quarter of what you have lost in weight:

- If you have lost 9 pounds before hitting a plateau then stabilize it for 2 weeks before moving to the BOOSTER phase (page 239).
- If you have lost 22 pounds before hitting a plateau then remain at this weight for 5 weeks before starting your BOOSTER.

I am not saying you should eat more to keep your weight at a plateau! If your weight loss is progressing, keep it that way, continue following the ATTACK program and menus, and move on to MAINTENANCE (page 271) when you have lost 75 percent of the weight you'd like to shed.

My benchmarking theory applies to those of us who, all things being equal, don't seem to be able to progress to the next level of weight loss and, of course, to those who need to lose more than a mere 5 pounds.

Please keep in mind that since your body is an individual entity it might react differently to benchmarking: Maybe you will rebalance all the fluids, nutrients, and hormonal levels faster than someone else, or on the contrary, you might be on the slow side. Do not fret as this is beyond your control. You just have to accept it consciously and not feel demoralized if you are a slow benchmarker. Remember that those weeks will be nothing when you look back at your successful weight-loss journey!

To stabilize your weight during the benchmarking process (or plateau), just keep on following my ATTACK menus and fitness routine (see "Rules of the ATTACK phase," page 121), make sure you get adequate sleep, and manage your stress as you have been doing so far.

PLATEAU CHECKLIST

While we are enjoying the plateau for what it does to our mind and body we also need to make sure it has not come about due to our lack of commitment to the program. Take a moment to have a hard look at what you are doing and answer the following questions (to which the answers should be "yes"):

YUMMY NUTRITION

Am I sticking to my TDD every week?	❑ yes	❑ no
Am I following the ATTACK menus?	❑ yes	❑ no
Have I kept my portions the same size?	❑ yes	❑ no

EASY FITNESS

Am I doing my daily 30-minute walk on an empty stomach?	❑ yes	❑ no
Am I doing one hour of cardio per day?	❑ yes	❑ no
Am I doing five 25th-hour exercises every day?	❑ yes	❑ no
Am I doing two anti-cellulite exercises every day?	❑ yes	❑ no

MOTIVATION

Am I still motivated to lose weight?	❑ yes	❑ no
Am I constantly identifying and eliminating weight-loss saboteurs?	❑ yes	❑ no
Am I writing in my blog every day?	❑ yes	❑ no
Am I sharing my success on social media?	❑ yes	❑ no

STRESS AND SLEEP

Am I sleeping enough?	❑ yes	❑ no
Am I practicing abdominal breathing techniques?	❑ yes	❑ no
Am I getting enough daylight?	❑ yes	❑ no
Am I having enough fun in my life?	❑ yes	❑ no

If you answered "no" to any question, you might have found the reason your weight loss has stalled. Get back on track and see if the pounds start dropping again.

GOOD-BYE, PLATEAU. HELLO, BOOSTER!

We love our plateaus because they guarantee a long-term result, but we should learn when to extract ourselves from the embrace! So that you avoid the trap of staying at your plateau weight forever, calculate the date that will signal the end of the flat part of your weight-loss curve and the start of the

BOOSTER phase, following my formula on page 158. This date can be written on a Post-it note and placed on your fridge or on your computer.

Write your BOOSTER starting date here: _____ and turn to page 241.

TOP 10 THINGS NOT TO DO DURING A PLATEAU

1. STARVE YOURSELF
Yes, if you stop eating you will lose weight. But, you will also send your body into starvation mode in the process. This means that it will learn how to better store the few calories you ingest, slow down your metabolism, and make it increasingly harder to lose weight.

2. SKIP MEALS
Skipping meals because you are not hungry is one thing; skipping meals to reduce your daily calorie intake is a big no-no. By introducing frequent famine scares, you send your body the message that this might become a permanent state, hence that the rate of your metabolism should be slowed down for your survival. As we've seen in point one, this is not a healthy, sustainable weight-loss strategy.

3. REDUCE PORTIONS TO A BARE MINIMUM
Controlling your portions is one thing (and a healthy one at that); making them too small will, yet again, send your body in starvation mode.

4. TRY ANOTHER DIET
Stay focused on our program. I never said it was going to be miraculous. I did say, however, that you will learn to establish a healthy lifestyle and reclaim your body. Trust me. I have helped thousands of women. I know it is not always a walk in the park but stay committed. Stay focused. Eyes on the prize!

5. BINGE EAT

Feeling depressed when the scale is not your friend might send you diving right into a tub of ice cream. This self-punishment is simply a way to attempt to justify your apparent lack of results.

Also keep in mind that just because the scale is not showing a smaller number doesn't mean your body is not working for you. Enjoy the other changes to your body: You might not be losing weight but you might be toning your muscles and losing inches all over.

Give yourself a pat on the back for all those subtle, yet important, changes.

6. STOP EXERCISING

You may well feel down when you hit a plateau, but this doesn't mean that you should give up your fitness routine. On the contrary, you should get more exercise to keep your endorphin levels high.

7. STAY INDOORS

When things don't go quite the way we want them to, we want to burrow under the duvet. It is a normal animal reaction but not a healthy one. You need sun. You need to meet people. You need to keep your serotonin levels high, so enjoy life and celebrate the new you!

8. DRESS SAD

Plateauing means celebrating your new body, not getting depressed because you stopped losing weight for a short period of time. Reward yourself for the progress you've made with a new colorful top, scarf, or dress. Say no to dull, bland, shapeless, slouchy clothes as long as this plateau lasts!

9. DWELL ON PAST DIETS

You might be tempted to think that you are failing at my program. That when you hit a plateau on a previous diet, you just

Continued . . .

switched to another diet where you began starving yourself—so, you ended up with the (false) impression that you had broken through the plateau. You are NOT failing. It's important to be patient; it takes time to imprint a new reference point on your brain.

10. SURROUND YOURSELF WITH WHINERS

Easy to whine when surrounded by whiners, isn't it? Well, don't! You have nothing to complain about. Maybe a friend or two might ask you how well you are doing, and this might make you feel bad. Maybe. But you are stronger than any negative comments that might come your way. Who has lost the weight? YOU!

You are totally in charge and responsible for your success. Explain to your friend that you are benchmarking. You'll soon feel like the smart one, educating others against yo-yo dieting. Doesn't it feel good?

And no matter what happens, remember this:

- You are rewiring your brain.
- You are succeeding.

Because to arrive at a plateau, you had to lose weight in the first place.

STAYING MOTIVATED

If a benchmark ends up lasting longer than you are ready to accept, it might become difficult to stay motivated. To help my BootCampers remain on course to their perfect weight, I have devised a few challenges, which really do the trick. The whole idea behind this is to challenge yourself every single week by adding a little tweak to your diet, fitness regimen, or stress management.

Here is a non-exhaustive list that has shown to be highly efficient. I suggest you try this list first and add a few more challenges of your own until your body starts losing weight again.

- One week without rice.
- One week with 15,000 steps per day, rain or shine.
- One week with a smoothie every day for breakfast.
- One week with 30 minutes extra cardio per day.
- One week trying new grains and seeds such as teff or fonio, instead of rice, pasta, and so on.
- One week trying three new sports or exercises (such as Bokwa or new Zumba).
- One week with 4 cups of Sobacha per day (page 69).
- One week with hot or cold soup for dinner every day.
- Bedtime at 9:30 with a book (no electronics in bed).
- Three yoga breathing exercises per day.
- No looking at your social networks alerts and e-mails right when you wake up.
- Your idea of a challenge _____.
- And another one _____.

As you can see, those challenges are pretty easy to integrate into your life, but I guarantee that periodically incorporating them along your weight loss journey will help you stay engaged and move you toward your ultimate goal.

ATTACK MENUS

Here are four weeks of menus for the ATTACK phase, to inspire you to make the right choices. There are a few recipes you'll recognize from DETOX on the menu and, of course, I have added a few low-GL recipes to tantalize your taste buds!

I've made some suggestions for choices when eating out, but visit any restaurant you prefer. Check out the menu online and find out which dishes might fit the ATTACK criteria (for low-GL foods, see pages 135–138). That way, you can enjoy your meal out with the confidence that you are not breaking any rules.

Along with favoring low-GL foods (organic, where possible), you should start each meal with vegetable or animal protein, such as turkey or hummus; or with fiber (kale salad, soup); and keep sweet things for the end of the meal. This greatly reduces the impact of any sugar in the food, meaning the body stores less in the form of fat.

From this phase on, unless you are doing a BOOSTER or TD Day, you may enjoy one glass of red wine per day (two for men). Remember to drink three cups of Sobacha per day in addition to your morning cup. Finally, even though I'm not suggesting you follow a strict gluten-free diet here, feel free to replace bread with a gluten-free version.

DAY 1

BREAKFAST

Juice of half a lemon in 8 ounces room-temperature water

1 cup Sobacha (p. 69)

1 Sweet Buckwheat Crêpe (p. 74)

1 coconut milk yogurt

■ **Feast:** Pink grapefruit

LUNCH

■ **Feast:** Salad of grated carrots with a drizzle of lemon juice

Quick Tuna Salad (p. 189)

1 slice whole-grain rye bread

1 orange

SNACK

■ **Feast:** Apples

Handful walnuts

DINNER

Celery Root with Pears (p. 221)

1 small portion (6 tablespoons) Vegetarian Couscous (p. 201)

4 slices Parma ham

2 apricots

DAY 2

BREAKFAST

Juice of half a lemon in 8 ounces room-temperature water

1 cup Sobacha (p. 69)

1 Sweet Buckwheat Crêpe (p. 74) with 1 tablespoon raw honey

1 Raspberry Milk (p. 183)

LUNCH

Salad of chicory with 3 tablespoons chopped walnuts and Garlic Vinaigrette (p. 110)

Feta and Olive Pasta Salad (p. 85)

■ **Feast:** Seasonal fruit salad

SNACK

Celery with Roquefort Cheese (p. 222)

4 squares chocolate (your favorite)

DINNER

Spring mix with Lemon Vinaigrette (p. 110)

Scallion Omelet (p. 202)

■ **Feast:** Ratatouille Provençale (p. 103)

1 pear

DAY 3 (Turbo Detox Day)

BREAKFAST

Juice of half a lemon in 8 ounces room-temperature water

1 cup Sobacha (p. 69)

10 raw almonds

1 Apple Smoothie (p. 184)

LUNCH

Salad of baby-leaf spinach, apple, red cabbage, and artichoke hearts with Lemon Vinaigrette (p. 110)

Spicy Black Bean Wrap (p. 259)

3 prunes

SNACK

10 raw almonds

1 banana

DINNER

Watercress with Garlic Vinaigrette (p. 110)

■ **Feast:** Brussels Sprouts with Green Tea (p. 104)

1 veggie burger (your favorite brand), sautéed with button mushrooms in 1 tablespoon olive oil

1 banana

DAY 4

BREAKFAST

Juice of half a lemon in 8 ounces room-temperature water

1 cup Sobacha (p. 69)

1 bowl muesli (no added sugar) plus 5 almonds, 5 hazelnuts, and ½ cup soy milk

LUNCH

Steamed globe artichoke with 2 tablespoons soyonnaise

Corsican Wrap (p. 198)

1 apple

SNACK

Handful baby carrots

3 tablespoons Hummus (p. 111)

DINNER

1 slice Cherry Tomato and Goat Cheese Flan (p. 203)

Salad of baby spinach with vinaigrette of your choice

3 plums

DAY 5

BREAKFAST

Juice of half a lemon in 8 ounces room-temperature water

1 cup Sobacha (p. 69)

1 Sweet Buckwheat Crêpe (p. 74) with 1 tablespoon Strawberry Jam (p. 77)

2 oranges

LUNCH

3 Stuffed Mushrooms with Walnut Pesto (p. 204)

■ **Feast:** Tomato salad with fresh basil

1 (2-inch-square) piece feta cheese

10 gluten-free crackers

SNACK

10 raw almonds

2 prunes

DINNER

Grilled Mackerel with Melon (p. 205)

■ **Feast:** Steamed French green beans served warm with 1 tablespoon olive oil, a dash of sea salt, and pepper

4 squares chocolate (your favorite)

DAY 6

BREAKFAST

Juice of half a lemon in 8 ounces room-temperature water

1 cup Sobacha (p. 69)

Half avocado, smashed, atop a slice of whole-grain bread, toasted, and sprinkled with sea salt

1 Green Morning Boost (p. 73)

LUNCH

Salad of sliced beets with Lemon Vinaigrette (p. 110)

Grilled Chicken and Cheese Wrap (p. 198)

2 kiwis

SNACK

15 hazelnuts

4 dried apricots (choose sulfur-free version to avoid ingesting too many chemicals)

DINNER

1 large heirloom tomato, sliced, drizzled with 1 tablespoon olive oil and a dash of sea salt

1 serving Grilled Lemon-Garlic Shrimp and Polenta (p. 210)

4 squares chocolate (your favorite)

DAY 7

BREAKFAST

Juice of half a lemon in 8 ounces room-temperature water

1 cup Sobacha (p. 69)

½ cup steel-cut oatmeal cooked in almond milk with ½ cup
   fresh blueberries

LUNCH

Green salad with Garlic Vinaigrette (p. 110)

1 grilled beef burger with steamed broccoli, 1 tablespoon
   olive oil, and a pinch sea salt

1 slice whole-grain bread

■ **Feast:** Pears

SNACK

5 Brazil nuts

1 banana

DINNER

Broiled Swordfish a la Niçoise (p. 206)

1 handful cherries

DAY 8

BREAKFAST

Juice of half a lemon in 8 ounces room-temperature water

1 cup Sobacha (p. 69)

1 cup Savory Buckwheat Porridge (p. 77)

1 cup raspberries

LUNCH

Eat out: Italian restaurant

■ **Feast:** Minestrone soup

Tri-colored salad (arugula, endive, and radicchio)

1 slice vegetable-topped pizza (whole wheat crust, if
   possible, or even gluten-free)

SNACK

1 small whole wheat pita bread

2 tablespoons Hummus (p. 111)

4 squares chocolate (your favorite)

DINNER

■ **Feast:** Carrot and Ginger Soup (p. 189)

Basque Piperade (p. 208)

1 orange

DAY 9

BREAKFAST

Juice of half a lemon in 8 ounces room-temperature water

1 cup Sobacha (p. 69)

1 slice toasted, whole wheat bread drizzled with 1 tablespoon olive oil and topped with 1 mashed, ripe tomato and pinch Maldon salt

1 papaya drizzled with lime juice

LUNCH

Eat out: Fast food sandwich shop (because sometimes it's our only choice!)

6-inch whole wheat wrap with turkey breast, your choice of veggies, and Dijon mustard

■ **Feast:** Apples

4 squares chocolate (your favorite)

SNACK

1 pink grapefruit

10 raw almonds

DINNER

Poached Egg with Arugula (p. 211)

Carrots with Ginger and Soy (p. 223)

3 tangerines

DAY 10 (Turbo Detox Day)

BREAKFAST
Juice of half a lemon in 8 ounces room-temperature water

1 cup Sobacha (p. 69)

1 Raw Chocolate and Maca Smoothie (p. 185)

LUNCH
Caramelized Jerusalem Artichoke Hearts (p. 197)

2 slices wild smoked salmon

■ **Feast:** Seasonal berries

SNACK
20 raw almonds, plus 4 dried apricots (sulfur-free)

DINNER
Raw Pad Thai (p. 224)

Grilled halibut with 1 tablespoon olive oil, seasoning, and lemon

1 orange

DAY 11

BREAKFAST
Juice of half a lemon in 8 ounces room-temperature water

1 cup Sobacha (p. 69)

1 Parmesan-Buckwheat Crêpe (p. 75)

1 Green Morning Boost (p. 73)

LUNCH
Eat out: Chinese restaurant

Small egg drop soup

Stir-fried tofu with vegetables

½ cup steamed brown rice

■ **Feast:** Fresh pineapple chunks

SNACK

10 hazelnuts

1 banana

DINNER

Chicken Fricassée with Tarragon (p. 212)

Salad of baby spinach with Garlic Vinaigrette (p. 110)

4 squares chocolate (your favorite)

DAY 12

BREAKFAST

Juice of half a lemon in 8 ounces room-temperature water

1 cup Sobacha (p. 69)

1 Sweet Buckwheat Crêpe (p. 74) drizzled with 2 tablespoons agave nectar

■ **Feast:** Oranges

LUNCH

■ **Feast:** Fennel and Pink Grapefruit Salad (p. 190)

Grilled turkey or chicken breast

1 slice whole wheat bread

1 persimmon

SNACK

1 vegan yogurt (soy milk, almond milk, or coconut milk)

10 almonds

DINNER

Endive salad with Garlic Vinaigrette (p. 110)

Poulet Basquaise (p. 97)

■ **Feast:** Raspberries

DAY 13

BREAKFAST

Juice of half a lemon in 8 ounces room-temperature water

1 cup Sobacha (p. 69)

1 Buckwheat Crêpe (p. 74)

2 tablespoons Banana-Coconut Compote (p. 187)

LUNCH

Garden salad with Lemon Vinaigrette (p. 110)

10 gluten-free crackers

2 tablespoons goat cheese

■ **Feast:** Seasonal berries

4 squares chocolate (your favorite)

SNACK

1 Date Smoothie (p. 73)

DINNER

Tuna Rillettes (p. 213) with 2 small baked red potatoes

1 spring mix salad with Garlic Vinaigrette (p. 110)

1 pink grapefruit

DAY 14

BREAKFAST

Juice of half a lemon in 8 ounces room-temperature water

1 cup Sobacha (p. 69)

2 Apple Muffins (p. 187)

5 tablespoons Banana-Coconut Compote (p. 187)

1 orange

LUNCH

Provençal Halibut Wrap (p. 199)

■ **Feast:** 1 mesclun salad (or baby spinach, lamb's lettuce, or arugula) with choice of vinaigrette

4 squares chocolate (your favorite)

SNACK

■ **Feast:** 1 small bowl berries

10 raw almonds

DINNER

■ **Feast:** Vegetable Skewers (p. 227)

Petrale Sole Wrapped in Prosciutto (p. 214)

1 vegan yogurt

DAY 15

BREAKFAST

Juice of half a lemon in 8 ounces room-temperature water

1 cup Sobacha (p. 69)

¼ cup steel-cut oats cooked in almond milk, with 1 tablespoon honey and blueberries

LUNCH

Pizza Wrap (p. 199)

1 apple

4 squares chocolate (your choice)

SNACK

1 pear

2 tablespoons peanut butter

DINNER

Chopped romaine salad with Cayenne-Avocado Dip (p. 229)

Cinnamon-Almond Chicken (p. 215)

1 vegan coconut yogurt

DAY 16

BREAKFAST

Juice of half a lemon in 8 ounces room-temperature water

1 cup Sobacha (p. 69)

Chocolate Pudding (p. 188)

10 raw almonds

1 pink grapefruit

LUNCH

½ cantaloupe

2 ounces feta cheese, plus 15 gluten-free crackers

10 cured green olives

½ cup gelato (flavor of your choice)

SNACK

8 ounces vegetable juice (homemade or store-bought)

2 slices deli turkey

DINNER

Healthy Chinese Rice (p. 226)

Asian Salad with Soy Vinaigrette (p. 191)

1 Asian pear

DAY 17 (Turbo Detox Day)

BREAKFAST

Juice of half a lemon in 8 ounces room-temperature water

1 cup Sobacha (p. 69)

1 Parmesan-Buckwheat Crêpe (p. 75)

3 tablespoons vegan cream cheese

1 banana

LUNCH

Grated carrots, avocado, beet, and jicama salad with Garlic Vinaigrette (p. 110)

Greek Salad (p. 192) with a gluten-free roll or slice of bread

■ **Feast:** Apples

SNACK

2 slices watermelon

15 raw almonds

DINNER

■ **Feast:** Soup (cold like Tomato Gazpacho [p. 257] if the weather is hot or a hot vegetable soup if the weather is cold)

5 tablespoons steamed quinoa with Stir-Fried Tofu with Dijon Mustard (p. 93)

4 slices fresh pineapple sprinkled with coconut flakes

DAY 18

BREAKFAST

Juice of half a lemon in 8 ounces room-temperature water

1 cup Sobacha (p. 69)

2 slices whole wheat bread with 2 tablespoons peanut butter and 2 tablespoons Strawberry Jam (p. 77)

LUNCH

Caesar Chicken Wrap (p. 200)

1 handful cherries

SNACK

Handful of baby carrots or 2 stalks of celery

2 tablespoons Hummus (p. 111)

DINNER

Orzo Pasta with Ham (p. 216)

1 sliced heirloom tomato drizzled with 1 tablespoon olive oil and a dash of salt

1 cup seasonal fruit salad

DAY 19

BREAKFAST

Juice of half a lemon in 8 ounces room-temperature water

1 cup Sobacha (p. 69)

3 scrambled egg whites with mushrooms and ½ tomato

1 cup grapes

LUNCH

Sweet Potato and Shiitake Mushroom Salad (p. 193)

2 slices wild smoked salmon

1 banana

SNACK

1 cup raspberries

1 small pouch plain beef jerky (avoid the teriyaki kind as it is loaded with sugar)

DINNER

Pea Clafoutis (p. 228)

2 slices baked ham

■ **Feast:** 1 cup Tri-Color Fruit Salad (p. 113)

DAY 20

BREAKFAST

Juice of half a lemon in 8 ounces room-temperature water

1 cup Sobacha (p. 69)

1 large papaya

½ cup low-fat cottage cheese with ¼ cup gluten-free granola

LUNCH

Frisée Salad with Rolled Oats (p. 194)

1 cup cooked chicken

1 slice Pineapple Coconut Tart (p. 233)

SNACK

1 gluten-free bar (e.g., Kind Bar)

1 pear

DINNER

Zucchini and Feta Timbale (p. 230)

Shrimp with curry sautéed in 1 tablespoon canola oil

Baked Apple (p. 234)

DAY 21

BREAKFAST

Juice of half a lemon in 8 ounces room-temperature water

1 cup Sobacha (p. 69)

3 store-bought gluten-free waffles, toasted, with 1 teaspoon
nonhydrogenated margarine and 1 tablespoon honey

■ **Feast:** Pear

LUNCH

2 hard-boiled eggs

Baby Spinach and Strawberry Salad (p. 195)

■ **Feast:** Nectarines

SNACK

Orange Quencher with Mint (p. 186)

15 cashew nuts (raw, if possible)

DINNER

Mariner's Mussels (p. 102)

2 small red potatoes, cubed, sautéed in 1 tablespoon olive oil, with thyme and rosemary

Pineapple Carpaccio (p. 235)

DAY 22

BREAKFAST

Juice of half a lemon in 8 ounces room-temperature water

1 cup Sobacha (p. 69)

Raspberry-Coconut Smoothie (p. 186)

15 raw sprouted almonds

LUNCH

Seafood Salad with Lime Vinaigrette (p. 196)

10 gluten-free crackers

1 banana

4 squares chocolate (your favorite)

SNACK

½ cantaloupe

4 slices prosciutto

DINNER

Bacon-Roasted Brussels Sprouts (p. 231)

5 tablespoons steamed brown rice with 1 tablespoon shredded Parmesan

2 slices fresh pineapple

DAY 23

BREAKFAST

Juice of half a lemon in 8 ounces room-temperature water

1 cup Sobacha (p. 69)

3 egg whites, scrambled in a nonstick pan with 2 slices of tomato, chopped, and 1 scallion chopped

■ **Feast:** 1 orange

LUNCH

Crab-Cilantro Wrap (p. 200)

1 small baby spinach salad with sprouts and Garlic Vinaigrette (p. 110)

Handful strawberries

SNACK

10 hazelnuts

½ cup low-fat cottage cheese with 1 tablespoon honey

DINNER

Normandy Carrots (p. 232)

Flounder Piccata (p. 217)

1 pear

DAY 24 (Turbo Detox Day)

BREAKFAST

Juice of half a lemon in 8 ounces room-temperature water

1 cup Sobacha (p. 69)

1 Sweet Buckwheat Crêpe (p. 74) with 3 tablespoons unsweetened applesauce

1 banana

LUNCH

Hearts of Palm and Chicken Salad (p. 197)

10 gluten-free crackers

■ **Feast:** 1 apple

SNACK

½ avocado sprinkled with lemon juice

10 raw almonds

Handful strawberries

DINNER

Grilled Tilapia (cooked in 1 tablespoon olive oil, with a dash of jambalaya spices), served with the juice of 1 lemon

5 tablespoons basmati brown rice

Salad of shredded kale, beets, and black beans with Garlic Vinaigrette (p. 110)

1 kiwi

DAY 25

BREAKFAST

Juice of half a lemon in 8 ounces room-temperature water

1 cup Sobacha (p. 69)

½ cup steel-cut oats cooked in almond milk with 10 hazelnuts and a handful berries

LUNCH

2 Ham-Wrapped Macédoine (p. 218)

1 slice Banana Bread (p. 236)

1 cup blackberries

SNACK

Handful baby carrots

3 tablespoons Hummus (p. 111)

DINNER

Gluten-free pasta with 1 tablespoon shredded Parmesan and store-bought marinara sauce

1 veggie burger

1 nectarine

DAY 26

BREAKFAST

Juice of half a lemon in 8 ounces room-temperature water

1 cup Sobacha (p. 69)

3 store-bought gluten-free waffles, toasted, with 1 teaspoon nonhydrogenated margarine and 1 tablespoon honey

1 papaya

LUNCH

Pizza Wrap (p. 199)

Baby arugula salad with Lemon Vinaigrette (p. 110)

1 cup raspberries

SNACK

8 ounces vegetable juice

10 raw almonds

4 squares chocolate (your favorite)

DINNER

2 slices Honey-Baked Ham (p. 219)

1 small mashed potato

2 slices pineapple

DAY 27

BREAKFAST

Juice of half a lemon in 8 ounces room-temperature water

1 cup Sobacha (p. 69)

1 toasted slice whole wheat bread with ½ mashed avocado and a dash of salt

1 peach

LUNCH

Typical Parisian lunch: Grilled flank steak with steamed French green beans

½ cup low-fat cottage cheese with 1 tablespoon honey

SNACK

10 Brazil nuts

1 banana

DINNER

- **Feast:** Cucumber salad (thinly sliced cucumbers and red onion, sprinkled with fresh dill and apple cider vinegar)

Grilled turkey patty, cooked in ½ tablespoon olive oil and herbs de Provence

Vegan Chocolate Pudding with Coconut Cream (p. 237)

DAY 28

BREAKFAST

Juice of half a lemon in 8 ounces room-temperature water

1 cup Sobacha (p. 69)

Green Morning Boost (p. 73)

Quinoa Fruity Porridge (p. 188)

LUNCH

Caesar Chicken Wrap (p. 200)

Grated carrots with jicama with Lemon Vinaigrette (p. 110)

4 squares chocolate (your favorite)

SNACK

1 vegan yogurt

¼ cup gluten-free granola

DINNER

Veal Escalope with Mustard (p. 220)

Mashed steamed broccoli with 1 tablespoon nonhydrogenated margarine and a dash of salt

Fresh Fruit Soup (p. 238)

ATTACK
RECIPES

RASPBERRY MILK

SERVES 2

Here is a way to enjoy "milk" without the concerns related to dairy products, like lactose-intolerance, for example. Almond milk is easy to make, and is a fantastic source of good enzymes for your health. My son, who is a good test, adores it! With a touch of berries you get a healthy and really tasty drink!

1 handful fresh raw almonds

1 teaspoon vanilla extract (or less, if you prefer a less distinct vanilla taste)

2 tablespoons agave nectar or organic honey

1 cup raspberries

1. The night before, soak the almonds in a bowl of water large enough to completely cover the almonds (they will expand overnight).
2. In the morning, rinse and drain the almonds. Put in the blender with two-thirds (or according to your taste) their volume of water.
3. Blend until the liquid turns white and milky.
4. Filter the milk through cheesecloth in order to eliminate pulp. Discard the pulp. (I personally keep the pulp to make raw snack bars, but that's another story.)
5. Transfer the milk to a blender, add the raspberries, the agave nectar, and the vanilla extract and blend until smooth. Enjoy right away.

APPLE SMOOTHIE

1 cup almond milk (store-bought or use the recipe from
Raspberry Milk, p. 183)

1 apple, peeled and cubed

½ teaspoon cinnamon

½ teaspoon vanilla extract

3 ice cubes

1 banana

1 tablespoon honey

1. Place all ingredients in a blender and blend until smooth. Enjoy
   right away!

RAW CHOCOLATE AND
MACA SMOOTHIE

SERVES 1

I know this recipe calls for strange ingredients, but I find it interesting to challenge ourselves once in a while to tantalize our taste buds and stay motivated! In this recipe you can replace the raw chocolate powder with dark chocolate (80 percent cocoa solids), and you could easily just leave out the camu camu and maca powder. Camu camu is a shrub found in the Amazonian rainforest. Compared with oranges, this powder provides 30 to 50 times more vitamin C, 10 times more iron, 3 times more niacin, twice as much riboflavin, and 50 percent more phosphorus. Maca is a root belonging to the radish family. It is packed with antioxidants and contains 7 essential amino acids. In short, it is really good for us!

1 cup almond milk (store bought or see Raspberry Milk recipe p. 183)

1 banana

½ teaspoon vanilla extract

1 teaspoon agave nectar

1 tablespoon maca powder (preferably organic)

1 teaspoon camu camu (available in organic health food stores)

1 tablespoon raw chocolate powder, or 80 percent dark chocolate, finely chopped

1. Place all ingredients in the blender and pulse until smooth. Pour into a glass and enjoy right away.

ORANGE QUENCHER WITH MINT

SERVES 1

2 oranges

4 fresh mint leaves, or more, to taste

6 ice cubes

1. Juice the oranges.
2. Place the freshly squeezed orange juice, mint leaves (or more if you prefer), and the ice cubes in a blender and blend until smooth. Enjoy this vitamin-loaded drink!

RASPBERRY-COCONUT SMOOTHIE

SERVES 1

2 handfuls raspberries (preferably frozen)

½ teaspoon vanilla extract

1 tablespoon almond butter (fresh, if possible)

1 cup water

2 tablespoons grated coconut (fresh or dried)

1 teaspoon agave nectar or organic honey (optional)

1. Place all the ingredients in a blender and pulse until well blended. Enjoy!

BANANA-COCONUT COMPOTE

SERVES 4

10 small organic Golden Delicious apples

2 small very ripe organic bananas

1 cup water

Juice of 1 lemon

1 vanilla bean pod, halved and seeds scraped

3 tablespoons grated coconut, unsweetened if possible

1 tablespoon thyme honey (or any other honey)

1. Peel the apples and cut into chunks. Place the apples and bananas in a medium saucepan with the water, lemon juice, vanilla seeds and pulp, coconut, and honey, and cook over low heat until the apples are quite tender.
2. Crush with a fork and serve warm.

APPLE MUFFINS

SERVES 4

1 egg

1 (8-oz.) container soy vanilla yogurt

¼ cup vegan sour cream

1 cup gluten-free flour

2 teaspoons baking powder

2 apples

⅓ cup crushed almonds

1. Preheat the oven to 350°F. Line 4 cups of a muffin tin with paper liners, and set aside.
2. Beat together the egg, yogurt, sour cream, flour, and baking powder.
3. Peel apples and shred. Add, with the almonds, to the mixture.
4. Mix well and pour into prepared muffin cups. Bake for 30 minutes or until golden and toothpick inserted comes out clean.

CHOCOLATE PUDDING

SERVES 4

2 cups almond milk

3.5 ounces dark baking chocolate

3 tablespoons brown sugar

1 packet powdered agar-agar (½ teaspoon)

1 teaspoon ginger powder (you can use cinnamon or orange zest for a unique twist)

1. In a heavy saucepan, slowly heat almond milk over medium heat. Add the chocolate and the sugar. The chocolate should melt, but the milk should not come to a boil.
2. When the chocolate is completely melted, add the agar-agar and the ginger. Raise the heat and bring mixture to a boil for 1 minute.
3. Pour into ramekins and refrigerate for 2 hours. Serve chilled.

QUINOA FRUITY PORRIDGE

SERVES 1

¼ cup quinoa

1 cup almond milk

½ teaspoon cinnamon

1 tablespoon honey

1 cup berries

1. Cook quinoa in milk according to instructions on package. Pour into a serving bowl.
2. Stir in cinnamon and honey. Mix well, top with berries, and enjoy!

CARROT AND GINGER SOUP

SERVES 4

1½ pounds carrots, peeled and sliced

1 onion, peeled and sliced

2 tablespoons olive oil

Salt and freshly ground black pepper, to taste

1 teaspoon ground ginger

3 cups chicken broth

2 tablespoons vegan sour cream (optional)

1. In a pot, heat the olive oil over medium heat. Sauté the carrots and onion until tender, approximately 10 minutes. Season with salt, pepper, and ginger. Add chicken broth.
2. Let simmer for 10 to 15 minutes, then purée with an immersion blender. Add the sour cream, if using, and mix well.
3. Ladle into soup bowls and serve.

QUICK TUNA SALAD

SERVES 2

1 (5 oz.) can no-salt-added tuna, packed in water

3 tablespoons soyonnaise (vegan mayonnaise)

2 tablespoons balsamic vinegar

1 teaspoon capers

3 chives, chopped

Freshly ground black pepper, to taste

1. With a fork, mix all ingredients, making sure to break the tuna chunks into small pieces.
2. Enjoy right away or keep in the fridge for up to 3 days in a sealed container.

FENNEL AND PINK GRAPEFRUIT SALAD

SERVES 2

Fennel is rich in fiber and supports good intestinal health and digestion. It is also an excellent stimulant and can soothe rheumatism. Grapefruit is now known for promoting low cholesterol; in fact, eating one every day for a month may reduce cholesterol in the body by 10 percent. Remember, though, that pink grapefruit can interfere with some medications. Consult your doctor if in doubt. Orange makes a good substitute.

1 large fennel bulb

1 firm pink grapefruit

1 teaspoon lemon juice

Salt and freshly ground black pepper, to taste

3 tablespoons fruity olive oil

Flat-leaf Italian parsley, finely chopped, for garnish

1. Rinse the fennel and slice thinly. Set aside.
2. Peel the grapefruit with a sharp knife. Remove the membrane, separate into sections, and remove the pith over a bowl, reserving the juice as you go. Then place the grapefruit sections in a colander, placing the bowl previously used underneath, to collect any remaining juice.
3. Combine the fennel and grapefruit in a salad bowl.
4. Make a vinaigrette with 2 tablespoons of the grapefruit juice, the lemon juice, salt, pepper, and olive oil.
5. Drizzle over the salad and toss carefully to coat. Garnish with chopped parsley. Serve right away.

ASIAN SALAD WITH
SOY VINAIGRETTE

SERVES 2

2 cups spring mix

2 tablespoons sliced lemongrass

FOR THE SOY VINAIGRETTE:

1 tablespoon reduced-sodium soy sauce

1 tablespoon red wine vinegar

5 tablespoons canola oil

Salt and pepper, to taste

1. To make the vinaigrette, whisk together the soy sauce and red wine vinegar. Slowly drizzle the canola oil into the soy-vinegar mixture and whisk until well blended. Add salt and pepper to taste.

2. Divide the spring mix evenly between two serving plates and sprinkle with sliced lemongrass. Drizzle with soy vinaigrette and enjoy!

GREEK SALAD

1 cucumber, unpeeled, washed and diced

1 tomato, sliced

½ red onion, thinly sliced

10 black olives

2 ounces feta cheese, crumbled

1 tablespoon fresh oregano or ½ tablespoon dried oregano

Sea salt, to taste

1 tablespoon olive oil

1. Combine the cucumber, tomato, onion, olives, and feta in a salad bowl. Sprinkle with oregano and salt and drizzle with olive oil. Enjoy!

SWEET POTATO AND SHIITAKE MUSHROOM SALAD

SERVES 1

1 cup chopped romaine

4 shiitake mushrooms

1 cooked sweet potato, sliced

¼ cup feta cheese, crumbled

1 tablespoon Dijon mustard

1 tablespoon canola oil

2 tablespoons lemon juice

Sea salt, to taste

1. Place romaine in large bowl and set aside.
2. Heat a small nonstick frying pan coated with cooking spray over medium heat. Add mushrooms and cook until softened, about 4 minutes. Remove from pan and slice.
3. Add mushrooms, feta, and sweet potato to romaine.
4. In a separate small bowl, make the vinaigrette by whisking Dijon mustard, oil, lemon juice, and salt. Drizzle over salad. Mix and enjoy.

FRISÉE SALAD WITH ROLLED OATS

1 bag frisée

10 cherry tomatoes, rinsed and halved

1 tablespoon pine nuts

1 tablespoon rolled oats

1 small shallot, chopped

1 teaspoon chopped chives

FOR THE DRESSING:

1 tablespoon mustard

1 tablespoon soyonnaise

½ tablespoon vinegar

2 tablespoons canola oil

Salt and freshly ground black pepper, to taste

1. Place the frisée in a large salad bowl and add the tomatoes, pine nuts, rolled oats, shallot, and chives.
2. Whisk together the dressing ingredients in a small bowl and pour over the salad.
3. Mix well and refrigerate until serving time.

BABY SPINACH AND STRAWBERRY SALAD

SERVES 4

Spinach! This nutrient-rich, dark, leafy green provides calcium, magnesium, vitamin B_6 and several other phytochemicals that are still being studied for their cancer-fighting capabilities. Vitamin B_6 is indispensable for your body to be able to process magnesium. A lack of magnesium may lead to noise sensitivities; nervousness; irritability; depression; confusion; twitching; trembling; apprehension; insomnia; muscle weakness; and cramps in the toes, feet, legs, or fingers.

FOR THE VINAIGRETTE:

1 tablespoon balsamic vinegar

1 teaspoon Dijon mustard

1 tablespoon minced shallots

2 tablespoons canola oil

FOR THE SALAD:

2 fresh bunches spinach, rinsed, drained, and pat-dried

½ cup dried strawberries, sliced

1 cup dried apple rings or half slices

Salt and freshly ground black pepper, to taste

1. Prepare vinaigrette by mixing together vinegar and Dijon mustard in a small bowl. Add shallots, then slowly begin whisking in the oil until well blended.
2. Put spinach in a large salad bowl. Add all but 1 tablespoon of the vinaigrette.
3. Top with dried strawberries and dried apples and drizzle remaining dressing on top.

VARIATION: As a blue cheese lover, I sometimes add blue cheese to this salad (just a tiny bit).

SEAFOOD SALAD WITH
LIME VINAIGRETTE

SERVES 2

3 tablespoons canola oil

8 shrimp, peeled, deveined, tails off

4 scallops

8 calamari rings

2 tablespoons soy sauce

FOR THE VINAIGRETTE:

1 tablespoon Dijon mustard

Juice of 2 limes

1 teaspoon tarragon

Sea salt and freshly ground black pepper, to taste

6 large romaine leaves, chopped

1 tablespoon Pecorino, crumbled

1. Heat 1 tablespoon oil in a large skillet over medium heat. Sauté shrimp, scallops, and calamari until fully cooked, about 6 minutes. Before removing from pan, add soy sauce and scrape the brown bits. Set aside.
2. In a small bowl prepare the vinaigrette: Whisk mustard, lime juice, tarragon, remaining 2 tablespoons canola oil, salt, and pepper.
3. In a large deep dish, place the chopped romaine, add the seafood, Pecorino, and the vinaigrette. Mix well to combine, and serve.

CARAMELIZED JERUSALEM ARTICHOKES

SERVES 2

2 cups peeled and sliced Jerusalem artichokes

2 tablespoons nonhydrogenated margarine

Salt and freshly ground black pepper, to taste

1. Sauté artichokes in margarine over medium-high heat until tender and caramelized. Add salt and pepper, to taste. Serve warm.

HEARTS OF PALM AND CHICKEN SALAD

SERVES 4

FOR THE DRESSING:

3 tablespoons soyonnaise

2 tablespoons red wine vinegar

2 tablespoons canola oil

Salt and pepper, to taste

FOR THE SALAD:

1 pound hearts of palm, drained and sliced

1 (8-oz.) can corn, drained and rinsed

8 ounces cherry tomatoes, quartered

12 black olives, pitted, quartered

10 ounces chicken breast, cooked and cubed

Parsley sprigs, for garnish

1. Whisk the dressing ingredients together in a large salad bowl. Add the hearts of palm, corn, cherry tomatoes, olives, and chicken. Toss carefully so as not to crush the hearts of palm. Garnish with the parsley.
2. If you have leftover salad, refrigerate it—it will be just as tasty the next day.

CORSICAN WRAP

SERVES 1

This is a recipe that brings me back to my sunny Mediterranean island!

1 whole wheat wrap

2 tablespoons soyonnaise

1 ounce feta cheese, crumbled

½ ripe tomato, finely chopped

2 tablespoons slivered almonds

½ red onion, thinly sliced

½ cup cooked chicken, chopped in small pieces

1 teaspoon herbs de Provence

Pepper, to taste

1. Spread the soyonnaise on the wrap, then add the feta cheese, tomato, almonds, onions, and chicken. Srinkle with the herbs and pepper. Roll and enjoy!

GRILLED CHICKEN AND CHEESE WRAP

SERVES 1

2 slices provolone

1 whole wheat wrap

1 cup baby arugula

½ cup cooked chicken, thinly sliced

1 teaspoon rosemary

1. Place the cheese slices on the wrap, then add the baby arugula and the chicken. Sprinkle with rosemary. Roll the wrap and heat for 1 minute on each side in a skillet on medium heat, or heat for 45 seconds in the microwave on high, just enough to melt the cheese and heat the meat through.

PROVENÇAL HALIBUT WRAP

SERVES 1

1 corn tortilla

2 tablespoons Baba Ganoush (p. 339)

1 halibut fillet, grilled or steamed, coarsely mashed

1 tablespoon slivered almonds

½ cucumber, peeled and julienned thinly

1 teaspoon lemon juice

1. Spread Baba Ganoush on the tortilla, and then add the halibut, almonds, and cucumber. Drizzle with the lemon juice, roll, and enjoy!

PIZZA WRAP

SERVES 1

Yum! The taste without the fat!

2 tablespoons marinara sauce

1 wrap

4 button mushrooms, thinly sliced

4 green olives, pitted, halved

1 teaspoon tarragon

2 fresh basil leaves

1 teaspoon olive oil

1 tablespoon shredded Parmesan

Freshly ground black pepper, to taste

1. Spread marinara sauce on wrap. Add mushrooms, olives, tarragon, and basil. Top with a sprinkle of Parmesan, a drizzle of olive oil, and pepper to taste. Roll and heat for 30 seconds in the microwave, if desired.

CAESAR CHICKEN WRAP

SERVES 1

2 tablespoons soyonnaise

1 corn tortilla

½ cup cooked chicken, diced

1 tablespoon shredded Parmesan

3 croutons, crushed

2 anchovy fillets

4 leaves romaine, shredded

1. Spread the soyonnaise on the tortilla. Add chicken, Parmesan, crushed croutons, anchovies, and romaine.
2. Roll and enjoy!

CRAB-CILANTRO WRAP

SERVES 1

1 tablespoon soyonnaise

1 whole-wheat wrap

½ avocado, mashed

1 small can crab meat, chopped in small pieces (do NOT use fake crab)

½ tablespoon fresh cilantro, minced

½ cup baby arugula

1 tablespoon balsamic vinegar

1. Spread soyonnaise on wrap. Add avocado, crab, cilantro, and baby arugula. Drizzle with vinegar, roll, and enjoy!

VEGETARIAN COUSCOUS

1 tablespoon olive oil

1 large onion (or 2 small onions), chopped

3 cloves garlic, chopped

Salt and freshly ground black pepper, to taste

1 teaspoon paprika

3 carrots, unpeeled, but washed thoroughly and chopped

2 zucchini, unpeeled and diced

1 small head broccoli, florets only

1 (15 oz.) can chickpeas, drained and rinsed

1 (5 oz.) can tomato paste

1 cup couscous

1. Heat the oil in a medium-size pot over medium heat. Add onion and garlic and cook until translucent and soft (about 6 to 8 minutes). Add salt, pepper, and paprika and enough water to cover the ingredients. Cover and bring to a boil.

2. Reduce heat to low so water is simmering, and add vegetables and chickpeas. Cook until vegetables are tender. Add tomato paste and simmer for an additional 10 to 15 minutes.

3. Meanwhile, prepare couscous according to directions on the package.

4. When ready, mound couscous on a platter and arrange the vegetables and the cooking liquid atop.

SCALLION OMELET

SERVES 2

5 eggs

Salt and freshly ground black pepper, to taste

2 ounces feta cheese or soy cheese in small pieces or grated

2 scallions, chopped in small pieces

2 tablespoons nonhydrogenated margarine

1. Break the eggs into a mixing bowl and whisk to blend for 1 minute.
2. Add 1 tablespoon of water. Season with salt and pepper. Add the cheese and the scallions and whisk together until combined.
3. Heat the margarine in a skillet over medium heat. Pour in the eggs. As the egg mixture begins to set on the bottom, lift one edge with a heatproof spatula and tilt the pan to let the uncooked mixture on top flow underneath. Keep lifting edges of the omelet and tilting pan, working your way around all sides, until no more uncooked egg mixture will flow underneath and the top is just a little moist—about 2 minutes total.
4. When the omelet is fully cooked, fold it in half and serve with your favorite salad.

CHERRY TOMATO AND
GOAT CHEESE FLAN

SERVES 6

One of my brunch favorites!

1 pound cherry tomatoes

5 ounces goat cheese

2 eggs

4 tablespoons cornstarch

1 cup fat-free whipping cream

1 cup fat-free milk (or vegan alternative)

Salt and freshly ground black pepper, to taste

8 sprigs chives, for garnish

1. Preheat the oven to 350°F for 10 minutes. Rinse and dry the tomatoes. Dice the goat cheese. Spread tomatoes and cheese in a single layer in an oiled baking pan.
2. In a bowl, whisk the eggs and the cornstarch. Add the milk and whipping cream while whisking. Pour over the tomato mixture.
3. Sprinkle with salt and pepper, and bake for about 20 minutes.
4. Remove from the oven and sprinkle with chives.
5. Enjoy hot or cold.

STUFFED MUSHROOMS WITH
WALNUT PESTO

SERVES 5

This is a unique, raw-food dish, where all the nutrients of the ingredients are preserved.

> 10 fresh mushrooms caps (cremini or others)
>
> 10 tablespoons olive oil
>
> Reduced-sodium soy sauce
>
> Rice vinegar (you can also use apple cider vinegar or other vinegar)
>
> Salt and freshly ground black pepper, to taste
>
> 1 bunch basil leaves
>
> 10 walnuts
>
> 1 handful pine nuts

1. Remove the caps from the mushrooms and brush to clean.
2. Place the caps in a large bowl. Drizzle with 6 tablespoons of olive oil, soy sauce, rice vinegar, and some salt and pepper. Allow the mushroom caps to marinate for about 1 hour, stirring as often as you pass by the bowl. If you forget, no big deal; it's raw food, no need to stress out in the kitchen.
3. In the meantime, put the basil, walnuts, pine nuts, the remaining 4 tablespoons oil, and a pinch of salt and pepper in a food processor. Pulse as necessary, to achieve the right consistency. I prefer my pesto thicker, while some people like it thinner. Whatever suits you!
4. When the mushrooms are fully marinated, drain them and place them upside down. Stuff them with the pesto, and there you have it: a great appetizer, a starter, or simply a garnish to go with an entrée (kids will love it too!).

GRILLED MACKEREL WITH MELON

SERVES 4

This recipe might sound like a strange combination but it is actually a classic Corsican dish—extremely tasty and very healthy!

> 1 tablespoon olive oil
>
> 8 small mackerel fillets
>
> 1 teaspoon grated, fresh ginger or 2 teaspoons ground ginger
>
> Salt, to taste
>
> ¼ cantaloupe or charentais melon

1. Preheat the oven to 475°F. Grease a large baking dish with the olive oil and set aside.
2. Season the inside and outside of the mackerel fillets with ginger and salt.
3. Peel and cut the melon lengthwise into small slices the same length as the fillets. Place the melon inside the center of the fillets and secure in place using kitchen string or twine.
4. Place the fillets in the prepared baking dish, with the open side uppermost. Bake for 5 minutes, then check that the fish is cooked. If not, add 2 minutes at a time, but no more than 4 additional minutes total.

BROILED SWORDFISH A LA NIÇOISE

SERVES 4

A typical dish from Nice, on the Riviera Coast, for which you can find different variations. This is the basic one.

6 cups water

½ cup pearl barley

½ cup olive oil

2 cloves garlic, crushed

4 (6-oz.) swordfish steaks

⅓ pound French green beans, trimmed

1 cup cherry tomatoes, halved

1 tablespoon herbs de Provence

½ cup pitted black olives, halved

½ medium-size red onion, sliced

3 tablespoons fresh lemon juice

½ tablespoon chopped fresh thyme

1 teaspoon grated lemon zest

Salt and freshly ground black pepper, to taste

Lemon wedges for serving

1. Lightly oil a baking dish and set aside.
2. Bring the water to a boil in large pot. Add barley. Cover pot and reduce heat to medium. Simmer until barley is tender, about 30 minutes.
3. While barley is cooking, mix ¼ cup olive oil and crushed garlic in a deep dish. Baste fish with the mixture and let marinate until ready to cook.
4. When barley is cooked, do not drain, but add French green beans and boil for about 5 minutes. Drain. Transfer to a large platter.
5. Heat 1 tablespoon olive oil in a large pan over medium heat. Sauté cherry tomatoes for 2 minutes and add herbs de Provence. Add to the barley along with olives, onion, remaining 3 tablespoons oil, lemon juice, thyme, and lemon zest.

6. Preheat broiler.
7. Place swordfish steaks in prepared baking dish and pour marinade over fish (broil in 2 batches if the dish is not large enough). Place pan in broiler and cook for 3 minutes. Turn fish and cook for about 2 more minutes, until fish is opaque in center. To avoid burning check often and if fish is getting too brown, move to center rack.
8. To serve, place fish over barley, drizzle with remaining juice in pan, sprinkle with salt and pepper, and add the lemon wedges.

BASQUE PIPERADE

SERVES 6

The word piperade *comes from "piper," which means "pepper" in Basque. Eggs are often added to this basic Basque staple, which includes onion, tomato, and green pepper. The three ingredients are of the same color of the Basque flag.*

4 whole sweet red bell peppers

1 tablespoon olive oil

1½ yellow onions, thinly sliced

2 teaspoons smoked paprika

1 teaspoon chili powder

1 (28-oz.) can whole peeled tomatoes

10 cloves garlic, crushed

2 bay leaves

1 teaspoon sea salt

1 teaspoon fresh cracked black pepper

6 eggs

6 slices crusty, whole wheat bread, brushed with olive oil

2 cups puréed tomatoes

1 tablespoon agave nectar

1. Roast the bell peppers over a medium flame by holding them with tongs and rotating them directly over the flame until they are blackened and the skin is starting to peel. (If you don't have a gas stove you can char the peppers in the broiler for about 20 minutes.) Place the peppers in a paper bag and seal tightly. After 5 minutes, remove the peppers from the bag. You will be amazed by how easily the skin comes off. After removing the skins, core, seed, and chop the peppers.
2. Preheat oven to 375°F.
3. Heat olive oil in a large skillet over medium-high heat. Sauté the onions for 5 minutes. Add the spices and cook for 2 more minutes.

Add canned tomatoes, breaking them up a bit with a spoon, and the add the crushed garlic, the bell peppers, and the bay leaves.

4. Reduce heat to low and simmer for 25 to 30 minutes. Add salt and pepper. (This piperade mix can be kept in the fridge for 4 days, or frozen if you don't plan on using it all at once.)

5. Place 2 cups of the piperade mix in an ovenproof cast iron pan.

6. Using a wooden spoon, make small holes in the piperade, in which you will place 1 cracked egg per hole. Bake until the egg whites seem cooked but the yolk is stilly runny. This should take anywhere from 8 to 14 minutes, depending on the size of your eggs.

7. Serve with toasted bread. Some serve the piperade on the bread slices directly.

GRILLED LEMON-GARLIC SHRIMP AND POLENTA

SERVES 2

A typical Corsican dish; polenta (the French equivalent of corn grits) is a basic staple on my island.

1 tablespoon olive oil

½ pound raw shrimp, peeled, deveined, and tails removed

Freshly ground black pepper, to taste

1 clove garlic, mashed

Juice of 2 limes

2 tablespoons Italian flat-leaf parsley, thinly chopped

½ cup cornmeal, cooked according to instructions (see Note, below)

2 tablespoons water or chicken broth

1 lemon, cut into wedges, for serving

¼ cup feta cheese, crumbled

1. Heat olive oil in a large pan over medium heat. Sauté the shrimp for 4 minutes. Add pepper, garlic, lime juice, and parsley (and 1 or 2 tablespoons of water if it is too dry). Toss around. Set aside.
2. Put the cooked polenta in a small cooking pot. Add water and the feta cheese. Blend well. Place the polenta in a shallow dish and top with the shrimp.
3. Enjoy right away, with lemon wedges served alongside.

   NOTE: I like to substitute chicken broth for the water to give it even more taste.

POACHED EGG WITH ARUGULA

SERVES 1

FOR THE SHALLOT VINAIGRETTE:

½ tablespoon balsamic vinegar

2 tablespoons thinly sliced shallots

½ tablespoon Dijon mustard

1 tablespoon olive oil

Salt and freshly ground black pepper, to taste

1 egg

Baby arugula

2 tablespoons white vinegar

1 tablespoon bacon bits

1. Prepare shallot vinaigrette: Mix the balsamic vinegar, shallots, and mustard in a small bowl. When smooth, slowly whisk in the olive oil. Season with salt and pepper, to taste.
2. Mix dressing with arugula and place the salad mixture on a serving plate.
3. Fill a small, deep saucepan with water two-thirds of the way full and bring to a boil. Reduce the heat to medium and add the 2 tablespoons white vinegar to water. Break egg in a small bowl. When water has reached a simmer, gently place the raw egg in the water, being careful not to break the yolk. Cook until done to your liking, usually 3 minutes are enough. Gently remove the poached egg from the water using a slotted spoon. Place on top of the arugula salad. Sprinkle with bacon bits. Enjoy right away!

CHICKEN FRICASSÉE WITH TARRAGON

This is a typical central France recipe.

1 pound bone-in chicken pieces, skin removed

Sea salt and freshly ground black pepper, to taste

1 tablespoon olive oil

2 shallots, thinly sliced

½ cup dry white wine

1 cup chicken broth

1 medium carrot, peeled and thinly sliced

½ pound button mushrooms, brushed clean and sliced

4 sprigs fresh tarragon

1 tablespoon cornstarch mixed with 1 tablespoon water

¼ cup vegan cream

2 teaspoons Dijon mustard

1. Season chicken with salt and pepper. Heat oil on medium-high in a large deep skillet. Cook chicken until browned (approximately 10 minutes total). Remove from pan and set aside.

2. In the same pan, cook shallots for 1 minute, then immediately add the wine, scraping any browned bits from the pan. Reduce heat to low and simmer for 4 minutes. Add broth, increase heat to medium, and bring to a simmer over medium heat. Return the chicken to the pan.

3. Add carrot, mushrooms, and tarragon sprigs. Reduce heat to low, cover, and gently simmer until the chicken is tender and no longer pink in the center, about 20 minutes, turning after 10 minutes. Remove chicken from the pan and set aside, covering with a lid or aluminum foil to keep warm.

4. Remove tarragon sprigs from pan. Increase heat to medium-high. Simmer the cooking liquid for 2 to 3 minutes. Add cornstarch mixture and cook, whisking vigorously, until slightly thickened. Whisk in cream and mustard. Enjoy right away.

TUNA RILLETTES

SERVES 4

1 (12-ounce) can tuna in water, drained

2 ounces Greek yogurt

2 tablespoons fat-free sour cream

1 teaspoon whole-grain mustard

½ cup lemon juice

2 teaspoons capers

Salt and freshly ground black pepper, to taste

1. Place the tuna in a bowl and mash with a fork. Add the Greek yogurt and mix to combine.
2. Add the sour cream, mustard, and lemon juice, and stir well. Add the capers, season with salt and pepper, and stir again. Refrigerate for 1 to 2 hours before serving.

PETRALE SOLE WRAPPED IN PROSCIUTTO

SERVES 3

A fancy dish to make for your guests. They'll never guess you're on a diet! If you can't find petrale sole, you can substitute lemon sole, gray sole, or flounder.

3 petrale sole fillets, preferably wild

3 thin slices prosciutto

1 teaspoon olive oil

Freshly ground black pepper, to taste

Juice of 1 lemon

2 tablespoons balsamic vinegar

6 toothpicks or twine

1. Preheat the oven to 350°F.
2. Roll the sole fillet. Fold the prosciutto around the fillet to form a "belt."
3. Secure each rolled fillet with 2 toothpicks or twine and place in a roasting pan.
4. Rub with olive oil and season with pepper.
5. Bake for 20 minutes, or until fully cooked.
6. Deglaze the sole juice with the lemon juice and balsamic vinegar.
7. Place the fillet on a serving plate, remove toothpicks or twine, and drizzle with the sauce. Yum!

CINNAMON-ALMOND CHICKEN

SERVES 4

2 tablespoons olive oil

2 large onions, sliced

4 chicken breasts, cut into pieces

2 thyme sprigs

Salt and freshly ground black pepper, to taste

7 ounces fat-free vegan whipping cream

½ teaspoon cinnamon

2 ounces sliced almonds

1. Heat the olive oil in a large skillet over medium heat. Add the onions and sear for 5 minutes. Add the chicken pieces.
2. Add the thyme and season with salt and pepper. Cover and cook over low heat. (Add some chicken or vegetable broth if necessary.) When the chicken is cooked through, 8 to 10 minutes, add the whipping cream. Add the cinnamon and sliced almonds.
3. Serve right away!

ORZO PASTA WITH HAM

SERVES 4

10 ounces whole-wheat orzo pasta

1 tablespoon nonhydrogenated margarine

1 onion, sliced

1 large, thick slice ham, diced

Salt and freshly ground black pepper, to taste

4 ounces fat-free whipping cream or vegan alternative

½ tablespoons dry rosemary

1. Bring 3 quarts of water to a boil. Cook orzo according to package directions.
2. In the meantime, heat nonhydrogenated margarine in a large skillet over medium heat and sauté the onion until translucent. Add the diced ham and sauté for a few more minutes.
3. Drain the orzo pasta and add to the pan. Season with salt and pepper and mix well.
4. When ready to serve, add the whipping cream and the rosemary. Season with salt and pepper. Mix well. Enjoy!

FLOUNDER PICCATA

The classical piccata sauce from Italy is usually used for chicken or veal. But in France we like to adapt this sauce recipe to other protein sources; here, we use flounder, a flaky, very tasty fish.

1 tablespoon olive oil

2 (6-oz.) flounder fillets

½ cup dry white wine

1 tablespoon nonhydrogenated margarine

3 tablespoons lemon juice

1 tablespoon capers, drained (see Note, below)

1 tablespoon gluten-free flour

Sea salt and freshly ground black pepper, to taste

1. Heat olive oil in a large skillet over medium heat. Sauté flounder fillets for 1 to 2 minutes per side, until flaky. Remove from pan and cover to keep warm.
2. Add white wine and deglaze the pan. Add margarine, lemon juice, and capers. Reduce and simmer for 5 minutes. Add flour and stir continuously, until the sauce thickens.
3. Place one fillet per plate, cover with the piccata sauce, and enjoy right away!

NOTE: Be sure you're buying capers and NOT green peppercorns. They do look quite alike.

HAM-WRAPPED MACÉDOINE

Macédoine are small pieces of blanched or steamed vegetables such as green beans, carrots, turnips, red beans, and so on. You can use your favorites for this recipe.

1⅔ cups vegetable macédoine

4 tablespoons soyonnaise

1 tablespoon balsamic vinegar

Salt and freshly ground black pepper, to taste

4 oven-roasted ham slices

1. Combine the vegetable macédoine with soyonnaise and vinegar in a bowl. Season with salt and pepper, and toss well to coat.
2. Lay 1 ham slice on each plate. Spoon a little of the vegetable macédoine along the center of each and roll. Chill until ready to serve.

HONEY-BAKED HAM

4 thick slices of ham, about 4 ounces each

2 tablespoons raw honey

1 teaspoon nutmeg

1 teaspoon cinnamon

1 teaspoon water

1. Preheat oven to 320°F. Oil a baking dish.
2. Place the ham slices in prepared baking dish and cook for 15 minutes, turning once after 7 minutes. Remove from oven.
3. In a small saucepan, combine the honey, nutmeg, cinnamon, and water and cook over medium-high heat until the mixture begins to boil. Remove immediately from the heat and pour over the top of the ham slices.
4. Return ham to the oven cook for another 10 minutes.

VEAL ESCALOPE WITH MUSTARD

1 teaspoon nonhydrogenated margarine

1 (4 oz.) veal cutlet

1 tablespoon low-fat cream, or vegan alternative

2 tablespoons mustard

Salt and freshly ground black pepper, to taste

Fresh sage leaves, for garnish

1. In a frying pan over medium heat, melt the margarine. As soon as it is melted, add the escalope and cook until nicely browned on both sides. (The cooking time will depend on the thickness of the escalope—to be sure, check that the center is white.)

2. Reduce the heat to low and add the cream and mustard. Season with salt and pepper to taste, garnish with the sage, and serve hot.

CELERY ROOT WITH PEARS

SERVES 4

Celery root has a long and prestigious history of use, first as a medicine and then later as a food. It is valuable in weight-loss diets, providing low-calorie fiber bulk, and is an excellent source of Vitamin C. For these reasons and more, it should be consumed regularly—not just once or twice a year.

As for the pear, it is not high in calories and contains a concentrated amount of essential nutrients. Vitamins C, PP, and B, potassium, calcium, magnesium, phosphorus, and zinc . . . an amazing contribution toward your daily recommended intake of vitamins and minerals!

1 pear, unpeeled

1 large celery root

Juice of 1 lemon, plus additional for coating vegetables

5 tablespoons nonhydrogenated margarine

1 sprig fresh thyme

Salt and freshly ground black pepper, to taste

1. Rinse and slice the pear. Brush the celery root under running water and cut into medium-size slices. Rub the celery slices with lemon juice to avoid any discoloration.
2. In a large skillet, heat the margarine over low heat, and then add the celery and pear slices. Add the thyme and half of the lemon juice. Cover and let simmer for 30 minutes, carefully turning the celery and pears from time to time.
3. After 30 minutes, transfer the mixture to a serving dish.
4. In the same skillet, over low heat, add the remaining lemon juice and scrape the bits from the sides of the pan until the liquid is reduced. Drizzle over the celery and pear mixture and serve.

CELERY WITH ROQUEFORT CHEESE

SERVES 2

4 medium-large celery stalks

1 cup plain low-fat yogurt

½ cup blue cheese

Salt and white pepper, to taste

1. Slice the celery stalks finely, and remove any strings if necessary.
2. In a pot, blanch the celery slices in one inch of salted water for about 2 to 3 minutes (no more, in order to keep them crunchy). Drain and rinse under cold running water.
3. In a small bowl, mix the yogurt, blue cheese, salt, and pepper, until combined well.
4. Add the celery and toss. Keeps 3 days in the fridge.

VARIATION: Instead of slicing celery, cut into 2-inch chunks and fill with yogurt mix.

CARROTS WITH GINGER AND SOY

SERVES 2

Make sure you use organic carrots here. If you can't find yellow carrots, then just use regular ones.

2 tablespoons olive oil

1½ cloves garlic

1 teaspoon grated, fresh ginger

¼ pound regular carrots (preferably organic), julienned

¼ pound yellow carrots (preferably organic), julienned

Salt and freshly ground black pepper, to taste

½ teaspoon ground cumin

1 teaspoon soy sauce

1 small bunch Italian flat-leaf parsley, finely chopped

1. Heat the olive oil in a sauté pan over medium heat. Add the garlic, ginger, and carrots and cook until vegetables are tender. Mix well and season with salt, pepper, and cumin. Add the soy sauce.
2. Lower heat and simmer gently for 15 to 20 minutes, adding a little water if necessary and stirring regularly. Add parsley and serve.

RAW PAD THAI

A raw recipe that requires a lot of ingredients so make sure you decide to make this one when you have the time to shop and cook.

FOR THE SAUCE:

1 cup light coconut milk

½ cup almond butter

1 teaspoon minced jalapeno

1 tablespoon minced ginger

2 tablespoons nama shoyu (see Note on p. 225)

1 teaspoon red miso paste

1 teaspoon minced garlic

2 teaspoons lime juice

2 teaspoons chopped dates, pitted

⅛ teaspoon cayenne pepper

FOR THE NOODLE BASE:

3 cups shredded daikon

1 cup shredded kale

½ cup julienned red pepper

½ cup grated carrot

1 scallion, bias cut

40 Thai basil leaves

2 teaspoons chopped cilantro

FOR THE GARNISH:

Cucumber slices, bias cut

½ cup cherry tomatoes, cut in half

⅔ cup chopped teriyaki (or regular) almonds

Mesclun mixed greens, for serving (optional)

1. To prepare the sauce, place all the ingredients in a blender. Blend on high until the mixture becomes creamy and smooth. Taste, and adjust flavors if necessary.

2. Ten minutes or so before serving, dress the noodles: Place all of the prepared vegetables from the noodle base into a large bowl and toss with the prepared sauce. If you haven't already prepared your garnish, do this while the noodles are marinating in the sauce.

3. Fan out three of the bias-cut cucumbers on the edge of each plate, and if using mesclun, garnish the other side of the plate with the greens. Place the Pad Thai mixture in the center of each plate, and top with halved cherry tomatoes and chopped almonds.

4. Serve immediately!

NOTE: Nama shoyu is unpasteurized soy sauce. You can substitute regular soy sauce if you can't find nama shoyu.

HEALTHY CHINESE RICE

1 cup brown jasmine rice

4 cups chicken stock

1 cup fresh or frozen corn

1 cup frozen peas

4 lettuce leaves, chopped

1 cup cooked chicken breast, chopped in small pieces

1 egg, slightly beaten

Salt and pepper, to taste (if you can find Sichuan pepper it is even better)

1. Cook rice in the chicken stock according to the directions on the package.
2. 10 minutes before the end of cooking, add the corn, peas, lettuce, and chicken.
3. Continue cooking for a few minutes. If the mix becomes too dry add ¼ cup water. When cooked, add the egg and mix on low heat for 2 minutes or until the egg is cooked.
4. Serve immediately.

VEGETABLE SKEWERS

SERVES 4

1 pound zucchini, sliced ½-inch thick

1 pound eggplant, peeled and cut into 1-inch chunks

2 red peppers, cut into 1-inch pieces

2 green peppers, cut into 1-inch pieces

6 small shallots, peeled

Salt and pepper, to taste

½ teaspoon cumin powder

⅔ cup olive oil

Juice of 1 lemon

1. Place the vegetables in a large salad bowl. Sprinkle with salt, pepper, and cumin. Drizzle with lemon juice and olive oil. Mix carefully to coat all vegetables.
2. Skewer the vegetables, alternating colors. Grill, turning the skewers about every 3 minutes. The vegetables must remain crisp.
3. When serving, drizzle with a little more olive oil. Can be used as an accompaniment to fish, meat, or simply brown rice.

PEA CLAFOUTIS

Traditionally, "clafoutis" is a baked French dessert of cherries arranged in a buttered dish and covered with a thick flanlike batter. Here is a savory version of this delight with peas and cheese, sure to be loved by kids and adults alike!

1 cup fresh shelled peas or frozen

½ cup diced baked ham

2 eggs

4 tablespoons whole-wheat flour, or gluten free flour mix, or rice flour

½ cup plain soy milk

1 clove garlic, crushed

Salt and pepper, to taste

3 tablespoons shredded Swiss cheese or soy cheese

1. Preheat oven to 300 °F.
2. Divide the peas among five individual gratin dishes. Layer with the diced ham.
3. In a bowl, whisk together the eggs, flour, milk, garlic, salt, and pepper. Pour the mixture over the ham and pea mixture, dividing it equally among the five dishes.
4. Sprinkle each dish with shredded cheese and bake for 20 minutes.
5. Enjoy with a green salad!

CAYENNE-AVOCADO DIP

Here is a solution to considerably reduce the fat content in your salad dressing. The avocado allows the sauce to homogenize so that the water does not separate from the other ingredients, giving us a beautiful, thick dip. Yum!

1 avocado

2 tablespoons lemon juice

1 tablespoon olive oil

1 cup water

1 teaspoon salt

1 teaspoon pepper

Pinch of cayenne pepper

1. Mix all the ingredients to obtain a smooth mixture. This dressing can be refrigerated for up to 3 days.

ZUCCHINI AND FETA TIMBALE

SERVES 4

4 medium zucchinis

¼ teaspoon salt

¼ cup chickpea flour or other gluten-free flour

½ cup low-fat fresh cream

3½ ounces feta cheese

1 egg, beaten

1 tablespoon thyme

1 clove of garlic, crushed

Salt and pepper, to taste

1. Preheat the oven to 375°F.
2. Wash the zucchinis and remove ends. Grate the zucchinis coarsely and place in a strainer. Season with salt and mix. Let sit for at least 10 minutes, 30 minutes being best.
3. Drain carefully, pressing out all the liquid. Pour into a salad bowl.
4. Add the flour, cream, feta, egg, thyme, garlic, salt, and pepper. Mix well.
5. Oil 4 ramekins. Fill each ramekin with the mixture and bake for 20 minutes.

BACON-ROASTED BRUSSELS SPROUTS

SERVES 2

1 pound Brussels sprouts, halved

2 tablespoons olive oil

1 cup chicken broth

4 tablespoons dry white wine

1 tablespoon vegan whipping cream

2 tablespoons bacon bits

1. In a large skillet, on medium heat, sauté the Brussels sprouts in oil until tender, gradually adding the chicken broth so that the skillet is never dry.
2. When thoroughly cooked, add wine, scraping the brown bits. Add the cream. Mix well. Then add the bacon bits. Mix one last time and serve.

NORMANDY CARROTS

SERVES 2

1 pound young carrots, peeled, julienned

2 tablespoons nonhydrogenated margarine

1 chicken glacé (concentrated chicken stock)

3 tablespoons dry white wine

4 tablespoons vegan sour cream

Sea salt and pepper, to taste

1. In a skillet on medium heat melt the margarine and sauté the carrots until tender.
2. Add chicken glacé. If the skillet is too dry, add water, ¼ cup at a time, but no more, to avoid a soupy mix.
3. When the carrots are cooked add wine and deglaze the pan. Add cream and mix well. Season to taste with sea salt and pepper.

PINEAPPLE-COCONUT TART

1 ready-made whole-wheat pie crust

1 large fresh pineapple

½ ounce nonhydrogenated margarine

1 packet of vanilla sugar

⅔ cup shredded coconut

½ teaspoon ground ginger (optional)

2 tablespoons packed brown sugar

2 teaspoons vanilla extract

1. Preheat oven to 375°F for 10 minutes.
2. Peel and core the pineapple and cut it into slices.
3. In a large sauté pan, melt the margarine and sauté 8 slices of pineapple.
4. Sprinkle with vanilla sugar and let caramelize for a few minutes, turning the slices regularly.
5. Place the remaining pineapple, vanilla extract, brown sugar, shredded coconut, and ginger in a blender and blend to obtain a homogeneous mixture.
6. Pour pineapple mixture into a saucepan and heat over moderate heat to reduce for a few minutes so that the mixture thickens a little to form a compote.
7. Pour mixture into the pie crust and spread evenly.
8. Lay the slices of caramelized pineapple on top.
9. Bake for approximately 35 minutes.
10. Let cool and top with more coconut.

BAKED APPLE

1 large organic apple, washed and cored, but unpeeled

1 teaspoon brown sugar

1 teaspoon nonhydrogenated margarine

1. Preheat oven to 375°F.
2. Place the apple in a large ramekin. Sprinkle the sugar over the apple, making sure some gets into the core. Put the margarine in the core.
3. Bake for at least 15 minutes and up to 30 minutes, or until apple is wrinkled and soft.
4. Wait 5 minutes before enjoying to avoid burning your tongue; the flesh will be very hot under the skin.

PINEAPPLE CARPACCIO

SERVES 1

Whether it's hot or cold, I love making this quick dessert, which is done in ten minutes!

Pineapple is a superb source of fiber, vitamin C, and contains an enzyme which some say makes you lose weight since it "burns" fat. Maybe, but it only seems to work in laboratories.

Fresh pineapple

1 teaspoon orange flower water or vanilla extract

1. Peel pineapple and cut 4 thin slices per serving, using a mandolin to get the thinness required for this recipe.
2. Place the slices on a small plate and sprinkle with orange flower water or vanilla extract before eating.

BANANA BREAD

1 teaspoon baking soda

Pinch of salt

½ cup brown sugar (see Note)

1 teaspoon vanilla extract

1 egg, beaten

3 very ripe bananas, peeled and mashed

⅓ cup nonhydrogenated margarine, melted

1½ cups gluten-free flour (Cup4Cup works well here)

1. Preheat the oven to 350°F. Butter and flour a regular-size loaf pan.
2. In a mixing bowl, mix the baking soda and salt. Add in the sugar, vanilla extract, and beaten egg. Add the mashed banana and the melted margarine. Only then can you add the flour. Please do respect this order to get the best texture.
3. Pour batter in the pan and bake for 50 minutes. Check the center of the cake (a knife inserted in the center should come out almost clean). If this is not the case, put back into the oven for 10 more minutes.
4. Remove from oven. Let cool on a rack. Only then you can remove the banana bread from the pan.

NOTE: I've also made this recipe with coconut sugar, and it tastes amazing!

CHOCOLATE PUDDING WITH COCONUT CREAM

SERVES 4

A rich vegan dessert, which I have been making since 2005, the year I discovered the famous coconut whipped cream!

⅓ cup brown sugar

⅓ cup raw cocoa powder

¼ cup cornstarch

3 cups coconut or almond milk (plain or vanilla)

4 tablespoons nonhydrogenated margarine

1 teaspoon vanilla extract

FOR THE WHIPPED COCONUT CREAM:

1 can full-fat coconut milk, refrigerated for 2 days

2 tablespoons coconut sugar, or brown sugar

1 teaspoon vanilla extract

Dash sea salt

1. Put a mixing bowl in the fridge. You will use it later for the whipped cream.
2. In another large mixing bowl whisk sugar, cocoa powder, cornstarch and slowly add the milk, whisking until the texture is smooth.
3. Heat over low-medium heat, whisking constantly until the pudding thickens.
4. Add margarine and vanilla. Mix well and if the pudding has the desired consistency remove from heat and pour into small ramekins.
5. Set aside in the fridge.
6. To make the whipped cream: Take the chilled mixing bowl out of the fridge. Open the can of coconut milk. Do NOT mix the content as you need to pour out the liquid part (you can use it for one of my other recipes that calls for coconut milk). Scoop out the cream and place it in the chilled bowl. Add sugar, salt, and vanilla and whip until stiff like a regular whipped cream.
7. Place in the fridge and add 1 tablespoon of this mix on top of the chocolate pudding before serving. To get a more professional-looking result use a piping bag.

FRESH FRUIT SOUP

SERVES 4

3 citrus fruit tea bags

4 ripe peaches

2 pears, not too ripe

1 bunch of white grapes

1 vanilla pod, split in half

¼ cup brown sugar

Champagne sorbet or your preferred flavor

1. In a small bowl, infuse the teabags in 1½ cups of boiling hot water.
2. Dice all of the fruit, except the grapes, and place in a deep dish with the vanilla pod and sugar. Pour the hot tea over the fruit. Let cool to room temperature, then place in the refrigerator for at least 2 hours before serving.
3. Remove the vanilla pod and serve in soup bowls with a scoop of champagne sorbet or your favorite sorbet flavor.

BOOSTER

GOAL:

SPEED UP WEIGHT LOSS AND

GET A FLAT STOMACH

BOOSTER

► **FACT:** Even though we are doing our best, toxins creep back into our body. To put this right, we periodically need a 7-day deep cleanse that will reset everything so we can continue losing weight efficiently and healthily.

► **FACT:** It is possible to get a really flat stomach!

RULES OF THE BOOSTER PHASE
- We drink Sobacha in the morning plus 3 cups throughout the day.
- We drink lemon juice with water every morning.
- We eliminate all food containing yeast and incorporate yeast-busting foods into our diet.
- We avoid all foods as for DETOX, plus a few more.
- We keep up our fitness routine, as for ATTACK.
- We manage our stress with abdominal breathing exercises.

You did it! You completed the first 2 weeks of my program, the DETOX, with dedication and good spirit. You proceeded with the ATTACK phase and its weekly TD Day, and established your first benchmark. You have now stabilized your weight and need to get out of your benchmarking period; or, you are done with ATTACK but would like to reset your body before starting MAINTENANCE.

We are now ready to carry out a 7-day BOOSTER phase. You might find this week the hardest of my program because of the limitations in foods you can eat. The beauty of this phase, however, is that you decide on the precise day that you start your BOOSTER. Wait until you have the time to take care of yourself, and more time for food shopping and cooking because, yes, this phase requires time-investment. But, I assure you, the results will be worth your efforts!

Once you are in the MAINTENANCE phase, do the BOOSTER whenever you feel you have overindulged and want to get back on track, or if you want to flatten your tummy. In any event, never do it more than once a month.

WHY A BOOSTER?

This 7-day phase will serve three purposes:

1. Speed up weight loss: You might wonder why you need to do a BOOSTER. You have already made so many changes. You are eating better, you are doing your weekly TD Day, you are exercising regularly to tone your body as well as eliminate more toxins. The fact is that, even with the lifestyle you are developing, you are still exposed to stress, pollution, and junk food. And, guess what? Losing weight also produces toxins, which are released when your body breaks down fat stores.

2. Shrink your waist: This is the number-one concern of all women (and men) I have ever coached. We all want a flat stomach but sometimes, no matter what we do, we still have a little round tummy. You might think that, because of your body shape, you are doomed. You are not! This should be your go-to phase whenever you find your abdomen not flat enough for your liking.

3. Help you end a benchmarking period in the ATTACK phase and restart losing weight.

In order to achieve these goals, we will start a 7-day nutrition program to cleanse your body and whittle your middle, boosting your energy in the bargain. During DETOX we began to clean toxins from our body. Here we are going deeper, from cleaning to "cleansing." The "S" stands for SUPER, as in super clean and SUPER flat!

First, let's examine how yeast can make it harder to reach the goal of a flat tummy, and how eliminating it from our diet can lessen bloating.

A FLAT STOMACH AND THE YEAST CONNECTION

A long time ago, when I was carrying excess weight, I read studies on how an overgrowth of yeast in the gastrointestinal tract could have a negative impact on the figure. I dismissed these, thinking they were not based on scientific proof. But, as the years passed, I took the time to do more research. And upon the discovery that candida (*Candida Albicans*) was a major culprit, I found a way to gain a flat tummy.

We need candida to live. It is present everywhere in and on our body. But when it overgrows in our gut as a result of our lifestyle, it leads to inflammations, infections (the dreaded "yeast infection"), athlete's foot, itchy skin, mental fogginess, irritability—and bloating.

Together, we will target your candida levels to make the dream of a flat abdomen a reality. (Your levels should already be lower, thanks to the Diet, but with these new steps you will be truly impressed by the results!)

> ▶ **NOTE:** Very few double-blind studies have actually proven that there is a link between candida and a flat stomach. Most conventional medicine practitioners tend to dismiss yeast cures, such as the ones that follow. I have drawn my conclusions from interviews I conducted with complementary and alternative medicine (CAM) practitioners, integrative medicine doctors, and naturopaths. For just this once I will ask you to make up your own mind. Read around the subject (I recommend *The Yeast Connection Handbook* by W. G. Crook). Try it out. Following my guidelines won't hurt you and you might even witness a miracle!

WHAT IS YEAST AND WHERE DO WE FIND IT?

Yeast is a one-celled organism belonging to the fungi (mushroom) family. Yeast can be our best friend or our enemy, depending on the strain and quantity we harbor or use.

There are many kinds of yeast, from the one we use in our baking, to those we use to make wine, whiskey and beer, or the supplement we favor for its high level of B vitamins. In nature, we can find yeast practically everywhere: in the soil, on plants, in water, on the skin of animals and human beings.

Like salt and sugar, yeast is ubiquitous in our food. It can be found in the vast majority of biscuits, brioches, breads, pizza, food supplements, drinks, and sauces. Along with mushrooms, foods like celery also contain high levels of molds or fungi.

WHAT FEEDS CANDIDA?

Candida thrives on sugar, starch, molds, and other yeast strains. To put it simply, too much yeast in your gut can make you feel bloated. In the BOOSTER menus at the end of this chapter, we will make sure we do not eat any foods that might support candida growth.

EIGHT FOODS TO BEAT CANDIDA

1. **Garlic**: A 2013 study by the University of Maryland Medical Center reports that candida-prone people may help avoid infections by eating more garlic. So, over the 7 days of the BOOSTER phase, add one clove of crushed, raw garlic per day to your meals, where possible.

2. **Probiotics**: The live bacteria in the kefir and probiotic yogurt will crowd out the candida yeast and restore balance to your gut system.

3. **Rutabaga**: One of the most potent antifungal foods you can find. Try it in vegetable soup, as chips (with unscented coconut oil), or mashed.

4. **Coconut oil**: Touted as a miracle weight-loss supplement, this might not, in fact, be such a marvel of nature (some studies have shown evidence to the contrary) but it offers potent antifungal properties. It contains high levels of lauric acid and caprylic acid, which help prevent candida overgrowth, while supporting your immune system.

5. **Onions**: These offer antifungal, anti-parasitic, and antibacterial properties. Ideally, you should have onions every day. If you fear for your breath, add some parsley to your dish to counter the smell.

6. **Lemon juice**: Lemon juice has so many positive benefits that it's on the menu in every single phase of LeBootCamp Diet.

In terms of fighting candida, lemon juice stimulates the peristaltic action of your colon, increasing the efficiency of your digestive system.

7. Cruciferae: We've seen that Cruciferae are fantastic for detoxing (pp. 51–52). They are also very useful in the BOOSTER phase, as all cruciferous vegetables (broccoli, cabbage, rocket) boast isothiocyanates—compounds containing sulfur and nitrogen—which attack candida. However, they can cause bloating (see below).

8. Cloves: These contain eugenol, an antifungal essential oil that is extremely effective when ingested.

EIGHT WAYS TO BEAT BLOATING

1. Chew, chew, chew: The digestive process starts in our mouth, so the more time we take over chewing, the more time our saliva and its digestive enzymes have to get working. When food arrives in the stomach half-chewed, larger food particles pass into the gastrointestinal tract, leading to bloating.

2. No fizzy drinks of any sort: The air contained in carbonated drinks can get trapped in our digestive system, causing bloating.

3. No gum: Chewing gum can cause us to swallow air, which can then get trapped in our stomach. However, gum can be an ally when you're trying not to overeat ("Top 10 Weight-Loss Tips," p. 152).

4. Pass on the salt: Too much sodium can cause bloating, too. Watch out for processed and frozen foods that can contain more than 200 percent of your maximum daily allowance.

5. Control your portions: When we eat more than the size of our stomach (remember, it's the size of your fist), digestion takes longer and food ferments. So, try eating four small meals a day—even five, if this works for you.

6. Beware of gassy foods: Avoid foods like beans or cruciferous vegetables, which can lead to bloating with some not-so-nice social consequences. Cruciferae are excellent for attacking candida, but if you react to them in this way, stay away or take natural anti-gas supplements.

7. Peppermint or fresh mint tea: My all-time favorite. Enjoy it during your meals or any time you feel bloated for quick relief.

8. Don't drink while you eat: This dilutes digestive enzymes, causing food to take longer to digest, leading to fermentation and bloating. Ayurvedic medicine practitioners suggest that you avoid cold drinks while eating. Try warm drinks like green tea instead.

You now have all you need to start your 7-day BOOSTER, which will help you get back on the weight-loss bandwagon while working on getting a flatter tummy.

FITNESS ROUTINE

During this phase you will keep up with your fitness routine, i.e., at least 30 minutes of slow-paced activity (walking or swimming) on an empty stomach, plus one hour of cardio, two anti-cellulite exercises (pages 144–151) and five 25th-hour exercises per day (pages 42–46).

Of course, feel free to add more as you should have enough energy to be really active.

STRESS AND MOTIVATION

Since stress can cause bloating because of the reasons we have explored in DETOX, it is critical that you practice some of the breathing exercises I shared with you (page 38), on a daily basis. I practice mine first thing in the morning so that I can start my day with a renewed sense of purpose and a minimal level of stress.

And as for motivation, make sure you weigh yourself on the morning of the first day of the BOOSTER as well as measuring the circumference of your waist. And then DO NOT MEASURE anything until the end of the 7 days. On the morning of Day 8, when you get back to your ATTACK or MAINTENANCE phase, you will get a lovely surprise; trust me on this!

So, are you ready? Let's do it!

BOOSTER FOOD GUIDE

FOODS TO FEAST ON

In addition to the anti-candida foods mentioned earlier (garlic, probiotics, rutabaga, coconut oil, onions, lemon juice, Cruciferae, cloves), you're free to indulge in the following:

- Seafood
- Wild, small fish
- Non-starchy vegetables
- Low-sugar fruits
- Non-glutinous grains and seeds (quinoa, buckwheat, teff, fonio)
- Herbs and spices
- Sobacha and herbal teas
- Fresh green juices

FOODS TO AVOID

- Fizzy drinks (whether regular or diet)
- Processed food products containing additives that may be harmful
- Processed cookies, sweets, cakes, and ready-made meals
- Fermented foods like sauerkraut or kimchi
- All dairy[1]
- Eggs
- All meat (including poultry)
- Gluten
- Yeast
- Alcohol
- Carnivorous and predatory fish
- Non-organic fruits and vegetables
- High-sugar fruits

---

1 Kefir permissible on 1 or 2 days.

- Any drink containing caffeine
- Rich sauces and heavy foods
- Sugar products
- All foods containing high-fructose corn syrup
- Aspartame and other potentially unsafe chemical sweeteners (pp. 29–33)

BOOSTER
MENUS

Our BOOSTER phase lasts 7 days. During this time we will focus on cutting down on foods that encourage candida growth, and on increasing foods that reduce it. We also bring in as many metabolism-boosting ingredients as we can, such as spices and ginger.

If you wish to expand my menu suggestions, feel free to tap into the DETOX menus and recipes, or even recipes of your own, as long as you stick to our rules for the BOOSTER phase, namely: no gluten, no yeast, no dairy, no meat, and no alcohol. I do, however, allow kefir (cultured yogurt drink) on some occasions, as it is excellent for beating candida.

DAY 1

BREAKFAST
Juice of half a lemon in 8 ounces room-temperature water
1 cup Sobacha (p. 69)
Chocolate, Banana, and Quinoa Porridge (p. 256)

LUNCH
Your favorite Mexican restaurant:
Tortilla soup (without the chicken or the sour cream)
4 tablespoons guacamole
15 corn chips
1 banana (bring from home or pick one up at the local market)

SNACK

10 sprouted almonds

C-Boost (p. 254)

DINNER

Wild Salmon en Papillote (p. 260)

Turmeric Millet Pilaf (p. 266)

■ **Feast:** Apples

DAY 2

BREAKFAST

Juice of half a lemon in 8 ounces room-temperature water

1 cup Sobacha (p. 69)

1 Parmesan-Buckwheat Crêpe (p. 75) with 2 fillets of smoked trout and mustard

■ **Feast:** Oranges

LUNCH

15 gluten-free crackers

3 tablespoons Avocado Dip with Capers (p. 268)

10 cured olives (green or black)

10 sprouted almonds (Place almonds overnight in enough water to cover them. In the morning, drain and rinse.)

■ **Feast:** Peaches

SNACK

5 Brazil nuts

4 squares chocolate

2 tangerines

DINNER

Sautéed Shrimp with Bok Choy (p. 261)

5 tablespoons cooked quinoa

1 vegan coconut milk yogurt

DAY 3

BREAKFAST

Juice of half a lemon in 8 ounces room-temperature water

1 cup Sobacha (p. 69)

1 Savory Buckwheat Porridge (p. 77)

1 banana

LUNCH

Your favorite Japanese restaurant:

Soba noodle soup with seafood

1 wakame (seaweed salad)

1 bowl edamame (soybeans)

SNACK

5 Brazil nuts

1 plain vegan yogurt with 1 tablespoon raw honey

DINNER

Baby spinach salad with Garlic Vinaigrette (p. 110)

Fish and Shrimp Crumble (p. 262)

1 papaya

DAY 4

BREAKFAST

Juice of half a lemon in 8 ounces room-temperature water

1 cup Sobacha (p. 69)

Carrot Boost (p. 254)

1 Sweet Buckwheat Crêpe (p. 74) with 1 teaspoon
nonhydrogenated margarine and 1 tablespoon raw honey

LUNCH

Mache salad with halved fresh figs, pine nuts, and Lemon
Vinaigrette (p. 110)

3 slices smoked salmon

1 slice gluten-free bread

■ **Feast:** Apricots

4 squares chocolate (your favorite)

SNACK

5 walnuts

■ **Feast:** Pears

DINNER

Cucumber salad with Garlic Vinaigrette (p. 110)

Cod Fillet on a Bed of Tomatoes (p. 263)

5 tablespoons cooked kasha (roasted buckwheat)

DAY 5

BREAKFAST

Juice of half a lemon in 8 ounces room-temperature water

1 cup Sobacha (p. 69)

2 Parmesan-Buckwheat Crêpes (p. 75) with 3 tablespoons vegan cream cheese

1 pear

LUNCH

Open-Faced Tuna Sandwich (p. 258)

Baby kale salad with Lemon Vinaigrette (p. 110)

1 cup blueberries

SNACK

15 cashew nuts

1 banana

1 cup coconut water

DINNER

Beet Millefeuille with Raspberries (p. 267)

Garlic Scallops (p. 264)

Chai Chia Cream (p. 269)

DAY 6

BREAKFAST

Juice of half a lemon in 8 ounces room-temperature water

1 cup Sobacha (p. 69)

Peanut Butter–Banana Smoothie (p. 255)

LUNCH

Hawaiian Wrap (p. 259)

1 cup strawberries

SNACK

Baby carrots

3 tablespoons Hummus (p. 111)

1 cup blueberries

DINNER

- ■ **Feast:** Tomato Gazpacho (p. 257) (if the weather is cold, go for a hot vegetable soup of your choice)

1 grilled trout with steamed French beans

1 vegan yogurt

DAY 7

BREAKFAST

Juice of half a lemon in 8 ounces room-temperature water

1 cup Sobacha (p. 69)

1 buckwheat porridge cooked in almond milk with 1 tablespoon chia seeds, 1 tablespoon honey, and berries

LUNCH

Spicy Black Bean Wrap (p. 259)

10 almonds

1 handful cherries

SNACK

Watermelon and Strawberry Quencher (p. 255)

1 apple with 3 tablespoons almond butter (peanut butter is okay if more readily available)

DINNER

Baby kale salad with Garlic Vinaigrette (p. 110)

Honey-Glazed Salmon with Edamame (p. 265)

4 squares chocolate (your favorite)

BOOSTER RECIPES

C-BOOST

SERVES 1

I call this drink the C-Boost because it is an amazing source of Vitamin C!

> 4 kiwis, peeled (not too ripe, otherwise they won't go through the juicer easily)
>
> 1 pear, unpeeled
>
> 1 apple, unpeeled
>
> 1 small bunch baby kale

1. Put all the fruits into your juice extractor and start juicing!

CARROT BOOST

SERVES 1

This recipe takes a little more time than some of the other boosts because you need to peel the pineapple. But, I promise you, the results are outstanding!

> 1 large carrot, not peeled, but well washed
>
> 1 cup fresh cubed pineapple
>
> Half bunch Italian flat-leaf parsley, rinsed
>
> 1 pinch sweet paprika (Espelette pepper is perfect)

1. Put all the ingredients except paprika in the juicer. Add the paprika and mix well.

PEANUT BUTTER-BANANA SMOOTHIE

SERVES 1

1 cup vegan milk (almond, rice, or coconut)

1 banana (frozen is better; make sure you remove the skin before freezing)

2 tablespoons peanut butter (raw is better)

¼ teaspoon vanilla extract

1. Blend all ingredients and enjoy. If the weather is hot, add a few ice cubes.

WATERMELON AND STRAWBERRY QUENCHER

SERVES 4

1 pound seedless watermelon, cubed

⅓ pound strawberries, hulled

1 tablespoon lemon or lime juice

1 tablespoon sugar or agave nectar

½ cup water

1. Place all the ingredients in a blender and purée.
2. Strain this fruit purée to get a clear juice, and enjoy immediately. The mixture freezes well, so make a batch and freeze it to have on hand.

CHOCOLATE, BANANA, AND QUINOA PORRIDGE

SERVES 2

½ cup quinoa

1¼ cups almond or coconut milk

1 tablespoon cocoa powder (raw if possible or as high as possible in cocoa content)

Dash sea salt

1 banana (half mashed and half sliced)

1 teaspoon vanilla extract

1½ tablespoons raw honey or agave nectar

Pomegranate seeds for serving (optional)

1. Cook the quinoa in 1 cup milk according to the directions on the package. If you need more liquid, add some water.
2. Mix cooked quinoa with cocoa powder, salt, mashed banana, vanilla, and 1 tablespoon honey.
3. Pour into a serving bowl. Add the banana slices and pomegranate seeds, if using. Drizzle with remaining honey and remaining ¼ cup milk.

TOMATO GAZPACHO

Tomatoes are an excellent food for your health because they are rich in lycopene (an antioxidant), which gives them their beautiful red color.

4 large ripe tomatoes, peeled and seeded

1 red pepper, seeded

1 (5-inch) piece cucumber

1 to 2 onions, chopped

4 tablespoons extra virgin olive oil

Salt and pepper, to taste

1. Dice the tomatoes, the pepper, and the cucumber.
2. In a blender, combine all the vegetables and purée. I like my gazpacho a bit chunky but you can blend yours until it's smooth if you like. Add olive oil and salt and pepper, to taste, and stir.
3. Pour in a bowl, cover with plastic wrap, and refrigerate for 4 hours. Serve the gazpacho chilled.

NOTE: Some chefs use other ingredients, such as garlic, basil, lemon juice, green pepper, or a little Tabasco. Feel free to experiment and try any variation you like! You can also decide to peel the cucumber should you want the gazpacho less green.

OPEN-FACED TUNA SANDWICH

SERVES 1

Quick and easy, this healthy dish provides good omega fats, protein, and fiber—enough to leave you full until the next meal.

2 slices of gluten-free, yeast-free bread

1 (3 oz.) can tuna in water (see Note)

2 tablespoons soyonnaise

3 tablespoons balsamic vinegar

Onion powder (or chopped fresh onion), to taste

1. In a bowl, mix tuna, soyonnaise, vinegar, and onion.
2. Toast bread slices and cut each in half.
3. Spread tuna mixture on bread halves to create 4 small, open-faced sandwiches.
4. If you are packing this to bring for your lunch, do not toast the bread and keep the tuna spread in a separate container until you are ready to eat.

NOTE: When buying tuna, "no salt added" is best, to reduce the level of sodium in your diet.

HAWAIIAN WRAP

SERVES 1

1 veggie burger (use your favorite brand, but make sure it is gluten-free)

½ avocado, mashed

2 tablespoons barbecue sauce

1 large or 2 medium corn tortillas

2 slices fresh pineapple, cut in small pieces

1. In a nonstick pan, cook the veggie burger. Mash it coarsely.
2. Spread the mashed avocado and the barbecue sauce on the tortilla.
3. Top with pineapple and mashed veggie burger.
4. Roll and enjoy!

SPICY BLACK BEAN WRAP

SERVES 1

1 tablespoon soyonnaise

1 corn tortilla or gluten-free wrap

½ avocado, mashed

¼ cup cooked black beans, slightly mashed into coarse chunks

¼ cup thinly sliced red onion

1 teaspoon balsamic vinegar

1 teaspoon hot sauce

1. Spread the soyonnaise on the wrap or tortilla.
2. Evenly top with the avocado, then add the black beans and onions.
3. Drizzle with balsamic vinegar and hot sauce.
4. Roll up and voilà!

WILD SALMON EN PAPILLOTE

SERVES 1

This is one of my favorite recipes because of the omegas 3, great taste, easy preparation, and simple yet beautiful presentation. What more can you ask for?

> 1 salmon fillet, preferably wild
>
> 1 tablespoon tapenade, or 3 green olives, sliced
>
> 1 teaspoon whole-grain mustard
>
> 2 lemon slices
>
> 2 cherry tomatoes, halved
>
> 1 teaspoon olive oil
>
> Salt and freshly ground black pepper, to taste

1. Preheat oven to 350°F.
2. Rub the salmon fillet with tapenade and whole grain mustard. If using green olives instead, first rub with mustard and then lay the sliced olives atop.
3. Arrange the lemon slices and cherry tomatoes on top.
4. Sprinkle with olive oil and season with salt and pepper. Lay the fillet in the center of a sheet of aluminum foil. Fold like a pouch and place it on a baking sheet. Bake for 20 to 30 minutes, depending on the thickness of the fillet.

SAUTÉED SHRIMP WITH BOK CHOY

As you know, during the BOOSTER phase we enjoy a lot of seafood and since bok choy is one of the healthiest and most detoxifying veggies out there, it is making an appearance here as well.

2 heads bok choy or Chinese cabbage

½ pound small shrimp, fresh or frozen, sautéed

1 apple, diced

Juice of ½ lemon

3 tablespoons soyonnaise

Salt and freshly ground black pepper, to taste

1 tablespoon sesame seeds (optional)

2 tablespoons chopped cilantro (optional)

1. Rinse the bok choy and pat dry. Chop and place in a salad bowl. Add the shrimp and apple, and pour the lemon juice over.
2. Add the soyonnaise and salt and pepper, and mix well.
3. Garnish this salad with sesame seeds and chopped cilantro, if desired.

FISH AND SHRIMP CRUMBLE

SERVES 8

This dish is topped with a crumble, which makes it sound decadent but it is still BOOSTER friendly!

1 cup gluten-free flour (my favorite is Cup4Cup), or rice flour

1 cup almond meal

¼ cup gluten-free Scottish oatmeal

1½ cups cold nonhydrogenated margarine, cubed

Salt and freshly ground black pepper, to taste

4 thin salmon fillets, skin removed

3 tablespoons olive oil

1 pound peeled carrots, julienned (about 4 large carrots)

4 tablespoons vegan sour cream

8 scallops, cut in half if large

½ pound shrimp

1 cup dry white wine

4 dill sprigs

1. Preheat oven to 375°F. Spray a 9 x 13-inch baking dish with cooking spray, and set aside.
2. In a large bowl, using your hands, combine the flour, the almond meal, oatmeal, and margarine, and a pinch of salt to obtain a granulated consistency. Refrigerate.
3. In a nonstick sauté pan set over medium heat, sear the salmon fillets for 1 minute on each side. Set aside with its juice, if any.
4. In the same sauté pan, still at medium heat, heat 2 tablespoons olive oil and sauté the carrots for about 7 minutes until soft. Add the sour cream, and season with salt and pepper. In a clean nonstick pan, heat remaining 1 tablespoon of oil and sear the scallops for 1 minute each side. Set aside with their juices. Add shrimp to pan and sear for 3 minutes total. Put aside.
5. Layer the carrots, and then the salmon fillets, shrimps, and scallops in prepared baking dish. Add the juices (from salmon and scallops) and the wine. Top evenly with crumble. Bake for 25 minutes.
6. Serve hot with dill sprigs on each plate and with freshly squeezed lemon juice.

COD FILLET ON A BED OF TOMATOES

SERVES 4

2 large tomatoes

2 tablespoons olive oil

2 cloves garlic, peeled and chopped

4 sun-dried tomatoes, cut into small pieces

2 tablespoons chopped Italian flat-leaf parsley

Salt and freshly ground black pepper, to taste

4 cod fillets, fresh or thawed if using frozen

1. Rinse and dice the fresh tomatoes.
2. In a sauté pan, heat the olive oil over medium heat and cook the garlic 30 seconds.
3. Add the diced tomatoes. Cook for 5 minutes, and then add the sun-dried tomato pieces.
4. Stir and continue cooking on low heat until the mixture turns into a purée, about 20 minutes.
5. Sprinkle with salt, pepper, and some chopped parsley, and simmer the tomatoes for a few more minutes.
6. In another nonstick pan cook the cod for about 3 minutes per side.
7. Spoon some of the tomatoes onto the center of each serving plate. Place one fillet on top and serve right away.

GARLIC SCALLOPS

1¼ pounds scallops

4 tablespoons olive oil

3 cloves garlic, peeled and finely chopped

1 tablespoon thyme

1 teaspoon chives, chopped

1 teaspoon parsley, chopped

Salt and pepper, to taste

1. In a bowl, combine the scallops, olive oil, garlic, chives, parsley, thyme, salt, and pepper. Mix well. Cover the bowl and refrigerate for 1 hour.
2. In a nonstick pan, sear the scallops on both sides, over medium-high heat for 2 to 3 minutes; be careful not to overcook them.
3. Serve right away!

HONEY-GLAZED SALMON WITH EDAMAME

SERVES 2

1 tablespoon lime juice

½ teaspoon grated ginger (or powder if more readily available)

1 tablespoon reduced-sodium tamari

1 tablespoon raw honey

2 wild salmon fillets, skin on

1 teaspoon canola oil

1 scallion, chopped

1 teaspoon black sesame seeds

1 cup cooked, heated, edamame

1. Stir the lime juice, ginger, tamari, and honey until smooth. Brush the salmon fillets with the mix. If you have time, let sit for 30 minutes to 1 hour in the fridge. This will help the flavors develop.
2. Turn on the broiler. Lightly oil a baking sheet. Place the fillets, skin down, on prepared baking sheet. Place about 10 inches from the heat source. Make sure you baste the fillets 4 times while they cook. Depending on the thickness of the fillet, it should take 5 to 8 minutes to be fully cooked through.
3. Remove from the oven. Place on warm plates, and sprinkle with scallion and sesame seeds.
4. Add the edamame and voilà!

TURMERIC MILLET PILAF

SERVES 4

1 onion

1 clove garlic

2 tablespoons canola oil

4 ounces cooked millet

4 ounces cooked brown basmati rice

4 ounces soybeans or white beans

Salt and freshly ground black pepper, to taste

Turmeric, to taste

Paprika, to taste

1. Peel and chop the onion and garlic.
2. Heat the canola oil in a medium-size pot over medium heat and sauté the onion for 5 minutes. Then add garlic and sauté for 1 more minute.
3. Add the millet, brown basmati rice, and soybeans.
4. Stir and season with salt, pepper, turmeric, and paprika.
5. Let simmer for a few more minutes. Add water or vegetable broth to prevent any scorching.
6. Serve immediately!

BEET MILLEFEUILLE AND
RASPBERRIES

SERVES 4

6 tablespoons apple cider vinegar

½ cup water

1 pinch Szechuan pepper

½ teaspoon grated ginger (or powder)

1 teaspoon stevia

2 whole cloves

1 red beet, cooked and sliced

2 ounces red cabbage, finely minced

4 ounces raspberries, fresh or frozen

1. Pour the apple cider vinegar and water into a pot. Add the pepper, ginger, stevia, and cloves.
2. Bring to a boil and then let sit for 5 minutes in order for the spices to infuse.
3. Place the beet slices in a bowl. Drain the spices mixture into a dish, and pour the liquid over the beets.
4. Let the beets marinate for 30 minutes in this juice.
5. Drain the beets and save the marinade.
6. In a deep serving dish, layer the beet slices, the cabbage, and the raspberries.
7. Finish with a layer of raspberries and season with the remaining marinade.

AVOCADO DIP WITH CAPERS

SERVES 2

2 ripe avocados

4 teaspoons capers

Green peppercorns

2 teaspoons olive oil

1 pinch of sea salt, or to taste

1 endive, rinsed (optional, for serving)

1. Crush the avocado coarsely together with the capers and a pinch of green peppercorns.
2. Add the olive oil and the salt. But remember to salt slightly because the capers already contain salt. Mix well.
3. To serve: fill the hollow of an endive with this dip for a pretty appetizer.

TIP: To prevent the dip for turning brown, keep it in the fridge with the avocado pit. If you are transporting it to work for lunch then keep the pit in the dip as well.

CHAI CHIA CREAM

1 cup raw cashew nuts

2 cups water

½ cup raw honey

1 tablespoon cinnamon

¼ tablespoon powdered ginger

¼ tablespoon ground nutmeg

1 tablespoon vanilla extract

½ cup chia seeds

1. Put all ingredients but chia seeds in the blender. Blend until texture is smooth.
2. Put mixture in a large bowl. Add chia seeds and mix well with a fork, carefully separating all seeds (they tend to clump).
3. Pour into 6 small ramekins, keep 30 minutes at room temperature then put in fridge for 2 hours. Enjoy!

MAINTENANCE

GOAL:

STABILIZE YOUR WEIGHT FOREVER AND

LOSE THE LAST FEW POUNDS THAT REMAIN

MAINTENANCE

▶ **FACT:** An obese or overweight body is acidic. A healthy and lean body is alkaline or neutral.

RULES OF THE MAINTENANCE PHASE

- We do one Turbo Detox (TD) Day per week.
- We drink Sobacha in the morning plus 3 cups throughout the day.
- We drink lemon juice with water every morning.
- We pay attention to our body pH and regulate it by following a healthy diet and choosing the right balance of alkalizing and acidic foods.
- We follow the MAINTENANCE fitness plans, according to our level of fitness, moving up as we progress and squeezing in 25th-hour exercises whenever we can. We continue to challenge the body, never resting on our laurels.
- We manage our stress with abdominal breathing exercises.

We are now all set to start the last phase. Look at all the progress you have made since we first started on this journey together! You have educated yourself in nutrition and fitness. You now know the difference between the Glycemic Index and the Glycemic Load. You know how to enjoy your food without gaining an ounce. You have put a winning daily routine in place. All credit to you for your perseverance and your amazing motivation.

Since you are moving on to the MAINTENANCE phase, it means you have lost 75 percent of the weight you wanted to shed, as we can only stabilize and maintain your success once that is achieved. So, hats off!

TAKE YOUR TIME!

*I*F YOU launch into MAINTENANCE too early, you can say good-bye to your achievements because you won't have waited long enough to "benchmark" your new body. Undertake MAINTENANCE too late and your motivation might go down the drain. Timing is of the essence.

Let's refresh our memory. If you have reached a plateau during ATTACK, be patient and observe your benchmarking intervals—in other words, adjust your thinking so that your plateau weight is your new "heaviest weight" each time. Remember to include a weekly TD Day and you will hit your target, guaranteed! You can also add an extra 30-minute walk per day and, most important, make sure you regularly document what you are doing in your blog to better identify your "diet saboteurs," as I call them.

Check again that you are not repeatedly falling for a rich afternoon snack with your colleagues. Remember, two slices of cake means that more than 800 calories sneak into your diet. And you must know by now that 3,500 calories is all it takes to gain one pound of fat!

Have you followed my plan to the letter? Have you jumped directly from a plateau in ATTACK, to MAINTENANCE, without completing your BOOSTER? Do you take your morning lemon juice? Do you drink your Sobacha? In short, question yourself honestly, and very quickly you will find the culprits, eliminate them, and get back on the right track.

If you haven't lost 75 percent of the weight you'd like to shed, I compel you to kick-start once more your weight loss with a BOOSTER, before returning to ATTACK. Only move on to the MAINTENANCE phase once you've lost the 75 percent!

MAINTENANCE FOR LIFE

If you've succeeded and reached your 75 percent goal, then bravo! Now let's get started with the MAINTENANCE phase.

Why 75 percent?

You have read several times already: I am insisting that you do not move to the MAINTENANCE phase before you have shed 75 percent. You might think that you should have reached your goal weight before starting a stabilization phase for life. I agree that it does make sense. However, here are the three reasons why 75 is the magic number:

1. During MAINTENANCE and because we are working on your pH levels you might find out that your initial goal was not realistic and that at optimal levels (pH, glycemic, etc.) your ideal weight is the one you have achieved in ATTACK.

2. As you add one more twist to your diet with the pH component, whereby you learn how to stay as alkaline as possible, your body will slowly continue to shed more pounds IF you are indeed still a tad bit over-weight. However, if you are not, you will stay at your ATTACK level and will consolidate this weight. Consolidating means you will set yourself in a position to never regain the lost weight and it will be easy to maintain this weight forever, even with excesses once in a while.

3. Psychologically, too, this phase is intended to have a measurable outcome for you. Without a weight loss goal a phase easily becomes mean-ingless and you might not feel as motivated as for the other phases. I have seen BootCampers go wild with excesses during this phase before I set an objective like the final 25 percent. However, and you will quickly discover it, as you regulate your pH levels, as you keep the vast majority of your life changes in place during this phase, you will reach your perfect weight. The one you can easily keep forever.

What is the point in stabilizing your new weight? After all, we have already spent several weeks (or months) together, and you are lighter and full of energy. You might think that you could perfectly well stop right away and enjoy your new body.

I am the first one to acknowledge that it is very tempting to tell our-selves all is going well, the goal has been reached, and that we can man-age on our own. However, if the vast majority of dieting attempts are met with failure—where we regain all the weight lost or, worse, gain even more—it is very often because we don't take the time to underpin our weight loss. (Not to mention the fact that some diets are dangerous or simply ineffective.)

On the basis of evidence from numerous studies, I have designed LeBootCamp Diet to include a MAINTENANCE phase that lasts at least as long as your ATTACK phase, and which you then adopt permanently so that it becomes part of your new life.

Why so long? Simply for you to get used to your new body, so that it becomes the permanent "new you," and so that you're never, ever tempted to go back to your "before" body. The only way to achieve this is to learn how to maintain.

This phase will also serve to identify small problems that you might still face. (That's why I say that MAINTENANCE is the phase where you are going to lose the remaining 25 percent.)

WHY SHOULD WE LEARN
HOW TO MAINTAIN?

The importance of learning how to maintain has been proven beyond any doubt. A large-scale study by researchers from Penn State University (published in *The American Journal of Preventive Medicine* in 2013) concluded that regaining weight after a diet is not inevitable, since we now know how to stabilize weight indefinitely.

Most significant, the study also revealed that the methods required to keep weight off are *not* the same as the ones used to lose weight in the first place. According to the author of this study, Dr. Christopher Sciamanna (Professor of Medical and Public Health Sciences at Penn State College of Medicine), "Losing weight then stabilizing one's new weight shares similarities with love and marriage. The reasons that take you to the altar are different from those which keep you married in the long run."

The researchers interviewed more than 1,100 people who had lost and never regained a significant amount of weight. From these interviews, they identified thirty-six techniques for weight loss and maintenance. They then conducted a large national poll asking people who started with a BMI of greater than 25 (i.e., overweight) to confirm which of those thirty-six techniques were the absolute best ones.

One of the key findings was that successful dieters had followed a *clearly identified weight-loss program* (as opposed to little tips gleaned here and there)—like LeBootCamp Diet, for instance! They had also reduced their sugar consumption, had not skipped any meals, and kept fit following a philosophy of Easy Fitness.

The study showed that the four most successful strategies for stabilizing the new weight (not necessarily valid in the weight-loss phase) were:

1. Adopt a diet with an adequate protein intake (vegetable or animal).
2. Follow a simple but consistent fitness routine.
3. Reward yourself (sensibly) each time you reach a milestone.
4. Regularly remind yourself of the reasons why you don't want to regain the lost weight.

Does this sound familiar? That's because these points echo the fundamental principles of LeBootCamp Diet. That is why you can trust me when I say that my method truly works: It has been scientifically proven to do so!

As we've just seen, we need the MAINTENANCE phase because the techniques needed to stabilize weight are different from those we used to lose it. I am asking you to follow this phase faithfully. Your success depends upon your commitment to the program. So, keep up the great work. We are not quite done yet!

MAINTENANCE AND BODY pH

The conclusion of Dr. Sciamanna's study, which is a key reference in the weight-loss world, is that the main difference between dieters who remain slim their entire life and those who fall continually into the vicious circle of losing, then regaining weight, is their state of mind and their level of motivation.

That is why the fourth concept we are going to explore together, central to the MAINTENANCE phase, is the concept of body pH. Why? Simply because not only does an acidic body make it harder to lose weight, but an acidic body is a tired body, without energy or stamina, which in turn affects our motivation level. A poor pH balance also triggers a slowdown in metabolism. As we know, a healthy metabolism is one of the cornerstones of weight loss and its maintenance. So—we need to work on our pH to support healthy weight loss. Simple!

In the DETOX phase, we introduced the concept of detoxification; in the ATTACK phase, we learned how properly managing the glycemic load of a meal can help limit insulin peaks, which transform us into fat-storing machines. Now, in the MAINTENANCE phase, we will discover how handling our body pH correctly can help us stay on the path of healthy and permanent weight loss.

(In fact, since you began this program, you have been rustling up alkalizing menus and recipes without realizing it!)

What constitutes 70 percent of our body, is pure, has a neutral taste and a perfect pH? WATER! And that's what our pH should be, as well. Throughout my program we are working hard to come as close as possible to this ideal number. You will see how easy it is shortly.

In chemistry, the pH is a measure of the acidity or basicity of a solution. If the pH is less than seven then we say it is acidic and if it is greater than seven we call it basic or alkaline. Pure water has a pH very close to seven, which we also call neutral pH.

Why is 7 a neutral value? Just as we've seen for the glycemic index in ATTACK, the pH calculation is based on a reference value: that of pure water at 77°F.

PH VALUE	LEVEL
0–6.9	Acidic
7	Neutral
7.1–14	Alkaline

Although the pH of any solution can go from 0 to 14, when it comes to our body the range is from 5 to 9 with an average at 7.35 (for the urine pH). Although you can measure the pH of blood, organs, saliva, and skin, please note that we will stick to measuring urine. Why? Because it is a very easy and painless procedure and a pretty accurate way to get a good reading of the state of our body.

The urine pH of a healthy individual who feeds herself correctly will be between 6.5 and 7.5. Just to illustrate my theory, here are two extreme examples:

- A sedentary, obese person who eats exclusively processed foods and red meat will have a pH inferior to 7 and close to 5—so, very acidic.

- A slim, healthy, and active person who eats a balanced diet, with whole foods, will likely have a pH close to 7 (neutral).

Our body needs to be at a stable, healthy pH level simply for us to stay alive! Indeed, the value of our pH conditions a large number of chemical and enzymatic reactions, which allow our cells to fulfill their functions. The closer our pH is to seven, the better our organs can function. The body does not need to consume energy to regulate its acidity level and can focus on other problems. Numerous studies have shown that an optimal pH level equips the body to prevent certain illnesses and sometimes even fight them. This seems to be the case, according to some studies, for cancer, osteoporosis, some allergies, arthritis, and rheumatism.

When all is balanced, we feel better in our body, hence in our head, and we're at the peak of our vitality. Our resulting improved digestion contributes to a stable weight.

On the other hand, an acidic pH leads to the accumulation of acids in the tissues, causing inflammations, demineralisation, and high blood pressure. In turn, those conditions can lead to osteoporosis, rheumatism, cancer, kidney disease (since the kidneys have to work double-time to compensate for excess acidity), diabetes, and obesity.

Sadly, this list is not exhaustive since even a small pH fluctuation can lead to a multitude of consequences.

HOW AND WHEN SHOULD YOU MEASURE YOUR BODY pH?

It's very easy. You can measure it first thing in the morning by using pH strips (these are available at any drugstore).

To be in the healthy range the pH of your first morning urine should be at 6.5 or above. Since this pH has not been affected by any drinks, foods, stress, and so on, I like to call it your basal pH. If you are already at 7.3, you are doing GREAT and your basal level is simply perfect. Now you will need to make sure you don't bring it lower throughout the day by letting stress take over or by eating poorly.

If your basal pH is too low (under 6.5), you are acidic. This means you need to raise it by doing the right things: drinking alkalizing fluids, eating well, and managing stress as much as possible, to bring your pH closer to seven or even better, above. (It's better to be slightly alkaline, because the body can easily become acidic, so this gives us more margin for staying the right side of neutral.)

Ideally I would like you to test your pH every day, starting tomorrow in the morning (and if, like me, you like to go the extra mile, during the day and at night). By doing this you will have a clear understanding of whether you have a healthy basal pH, made acidic by the way you lead your life, or, if you have a not-so-good pH at the start of your day, which you are able to change to neutral or alkaline by doing the right things.

It is also very possible that your morning pH is perfect and that it stays that way. Indeed, we have spent a few weeks together already, so if you have followed my program to the letter, it is very likely that your pH is at a healthy level. If this is the case let's stay on the right track!

> **NOTE:** In order to keep track of your pH evolution I suggest you record it in the blog you have been keeping during our journey together.

WHY CAN'T MY HEALTHY BODY TAKE CARE OF ITS OWN pH?

This is a question that I hear very often, both from journalists and BootCampers. Let's look first at how the body regulates pH. Two major organs support body pH balancing: our lungs and our kidneys.

Lungs: If your body becomes too acidic (with a low pH) it will respond by hyperventilating. It transforms the ions responsible for the acidosis into carbon dioxide (CO_2) and steam. When carbon dioxide levels in the blood are too high, the lungs start hyperventilating in order to exhale the CO_2, thus regulating its pH.

Kidneys: When hyperventilation is not enough to eliminate excess CO_2, our kidneys take over and expel hydrogen ions into the urine, in the form of ammonia. This is what turns your urine acidic. If acid levels become toxic, the kidneys are able to raise pH levels by reabsorbing bicarbonate ions.

It seems that our body is well equipped to face any pH challenge. However, the way we live today—high levels of oxidative stress, a poor diet, and a sedentary lifestyle—can turn our pH levels chronically acidic. So, we need to support our body in order to maintain the correct pH level in the same way that our detoxifying functions also need support at the pH level.

HOW TO BOOST YOUR pH

THE PROBLEM: Lack of Oxygen

As we've just seen, the body uses breathing as a defense mechanism for balancing acidity levels. But do we truly take the time to breathe correctly and get as much oxygen into our body as we need? We lead increasingly sedentary lifestyles and are constantly exposed to pollution. We live in houses and office spaces that are overheated, over-air-conditioned, or poorly ventilated. This leads to a lack of oxygen in our system, which in turn leads to an increase of carbon dioxide in our blood. The result? Our body cannot ventilate itself properly, and is thus unable to eliminate acid effectively.

Increased stress levels have also been strongly linked to a lack of oxygen, since a stressed person may have a tendency to slouch, thereby compressing the thorax and diminishing lung capacity. You must have noticed it: When you are under pressure your breathing is so shallow that very soon you need to take a deep breath. This is concrete evidence that you don't have enough oxygen in your body.

THE SOLUTION: Get Your Oxygen Fix

Getting the right amount of oxygen into your body will have a hugely positive effect on your pH. Use these simple techniques to clear acidosis and reduce the feeling of tiredness:

Ventilate! Health professionals advise us to change the air in our house for at least 10 minutes per day to eliminate dust mites and other microorganisms in our mattresses. This also replaces some of the carbon dioxide you generate during the night, with oxygen. Open the windows at least every morning in each room of your house and once more in the afternoon if you work from home. Also, when you open the windows in the morning use this opportunity to do 2 minutes of intense abdominal breathing like we saw in the DETOX phase: Inhale through both nostrils while inflating your abdomen as well as your thorax, then exhale through the mouth while sucking in your abdomen and emptying your lungs as much as possible.

Breathing fresh air is stimulating because it helps increase the level of oxygen in your body, thereby reducing the excess carbon dioxide in your blood. If you want to see how powerful this technique is, stay in an unventilated office space all morning and you will see how exhausted you feel by lunchtime. Then, go out—jog, run, or walk at a fast pace, taking care to inhale and exhale fully. Just 10 minutes are enough to witness a miracle: Your energy is back! How impressive that only a 10-minute walk outside can restore your pH balance.

Move more! Beyond the regular physical activity one needs to perform in order to be healthy, make sure you get your daily walking fix. Remember my famous 30 minutes on an empty stomach? Keep it going and make it a habit for life!

Get taller! Adopt a good posture when you are sitting at your desk, driving, and eating—even when you are walking. Stand tall and gently rotate your shoulders and neck; open your upper body by drawing your shoulder blades together. This posture will not only protect your back and help increase your lung capacity, but it will also send your self-confidence soaring.

Go green! Take advantage of the weekend to take your family and friends to a park or the countryside, far away from the city, or at least away from polluted areas and main roads. Just enjoy the moment: far removed from the noise (less stress), with purer air all around (better for your oxygen levels).

Go even greener! It's a fact: Some plants are not only a great help in reducing the level of pollution in your house but can also purify the air you breathe. They capture carbon dioxide during the day and produce oxygen. Though you might have heard that they produce CO_2 during the night, in fact, plants actually absorb more CO_2 than they make and produce more oxygen than they absorb.

So, place plants everywhere in your house. Studies by NASA Phyt'air program (2007) and the Faculty of Pharmacy at the University of Lille, France (2011), show that the spider plant (chlorophytum comosum) has undeniable purifying qualities. In 24 hours, the chlorophytum plant can absorb more than 86 percent of the formaldehyde and 96 percent of the carbon monoxide in the air of a closed, average-size bedroom. It makes the air in our house more breathable and helps alleviate allergy symptoms.

THE PROBLEM: Stress

We know already that overwork, lack of sleep, and stress slow the elimination of metabolic toxic waste (as well as causing a lack of oxygen in our system). This has been proven to lower our body's pH, thereby inducing a state of acidosis.

THE SOLUTION: Move Toward a Stress-Free Life

Easier said than done, you might think. Though we do need to keep a certain level of positive stress, we also need to reduce negative (or oxidative) stress as much as possible since this speeds up our cells' aging process and considerably reduces our body pH.

Here are a few tips to help you achieve this goal.

Move! We know that physical activity increases the oxygen in our system. It is also proven that if you move regularly, whether by walking around the block, playing a game of sports with friends, or going to a group fitness class you can boost your morale and your energy levels. And if you consider the fact that you also burn calories in the process, you can kill two birds (or three, in this case) with one stone.

Breathe! Stress, exhaustion, pressure . . . there are so many situations where a little respite is needed. Practice my breathing routines (or "yoga breathing") regularly to help empty your mind and get energized (pp. 38–39). They will help reduce pressure, increase your oxygen levels, and bring a feeling of well-being (and hence a higher pH). Do these as soon as you feel you need them—better still, don't even wait for the point of no return; make yoga breathing a daily routine, just like brushing your teeth.

THE PROBLEM: Poor Digestion

Again, our busy lifestyle is the culprit here. We work farther and farther away from where we live. We cut our lunch break short to finish an urgent project so that we may make it back home in good time. Eating on the go is commonplace, as is eating at our desk—we don't even take the time to sit in a separate area. Enjoying breakfast with the entire family is an event so rare that we have to plan for it—a sad reminder of what our mornings have become: a race against time.

Worse still, we don't bother chewing our food (and chewing is such a critical part of the digestive process). Because we don't take the time to eat properly, our ability to digest deteriorates. Poor digestion leads to constipation (lovely!), bloating, and gas as well as toxic waste that our liver will have to work hard to eliminate. With all this going on, it's no wonder our body has no energy left to regulate our pH levels!

THE SOLUTION: Take Time over Meals

- Sit down for lunch: Avoid eating on the run, in your car, or standing in your office or at your desk.
- Allow yourself 20 minutes *minimum* for lunch.
- Chew each bite 5 to 7 times.
- Put down your fork between bites.

THE PROBLEM: An Unbalanced Diet

The modern Western diet usually contains too many acidic foods (too much animal protein, processed meals, ready meals and so on) and not enough alkaline foods.

The way we preserve, cook, and eat food can also have a negative effect on our pH balance: the overprocessing of grains; a drastic reduction in our consumption of raw fruit and vegetables; too much sodium; too many flavor enhancers, artificial colorings, texturizers, and so on. All of these contribute to an acidosis that our body cannot regulate if it becomes too frequent.

THE SOLUTION: Improve Your Diet, Step-by-Step

This is certainly the most important factor toward improving your pH, but any dietary changes should be done at your own pace. I don't recommend radically altering all your eating habits because that is the best way to feel discouraged by the mountain of things you need to change. Take it one step at a time and you will win this battle!

MAINTENANCE FOOD GUIDE

ALKALIZING FOODS

- All green vegetables, raw or cooked (asparagus; cruciferous vegetables such as broccoli, cabbage, kale; cucumbers; green beans; peas; salad leaves), eggplants, carrots, celery, potatoes, sweet potatoes, olives
- All fruits: apples, bananas, dates, grapes, lemons, kiwis, melons, oranges, peaches, pears, pineapples, raspberries, strawberries, tomatoes, blueberries, plums
- Raw, unpasteurized milk (preferably sheep's or goat's), homemade plain yogurt, cottage cheese, eggs
- Sobacha (p. 69), green tea, water
- LeBootCamp alkalizing drinks (p. 316)
- Sprouted seeds and nuts, chestnuts, millet, soy, tofu, flaxseed,
- Apple cider vinegar, cinnamon, curry powder, garlic, ginger, onions, herbs, miso, mustard, sea salt, tamari
- Stevia, xylitol, seaweeds, bee pollen

ACIDIFYING FOODS

- Legumes, sweet corn, winter squash
- Fish (though wild Alaskan salmon is the least acidifying), seafood, all meats
- All other dairy
- Coffee, black tea, alcohol, carbonated drinks
- Prunes, canned and glazed fruits
- Nonsprouted nuts and seeds
- All grains
- Ketchup, pepper, white vinegar
- Bread, pastries, pasta
- Sugar, sucralose, corn syrup, carob, cocoa

BEWARE OF DEMONIZING
ACIDIFYING FOODS

Even though I recommend reducing acidifying foods to a minimum, it is essential—critical, even—that we don't get carried away and demonize acidifying foods. Indeed, just because a food is acidifying does not make it a poison. In the same way as with the so-called "good" and "bad" cholesterols, what matters is to strike the right balance between alkalizing and acidifying foods.

In a well-balanced diet, one should never, ever exclude entire food groups. It's all about balance and reducing the percentage of acidifying foods in our diet. This healthy strategy will help us stay on the right track without becoming obsessive about counting points, calories, and ounces; or depressed because we have to remove some of our favorite foods from our life.

For instance, whole-grain bread is acidifying. However, because it contains important ingredients that are good for us such as fiber, magnesium, and vitamin B_2, it should still be included in a healthy diet. Cereal products and high-protein foods, like meat and some cheeses, are very acidic. That is the reason why people who follow a high-protein diet have an acidic body, acidic-smelling sweat, and noxious breath. The adverse effects of such a diet on the kidney system have been demonstrated time and time again.

You may be surprised to see lemons in the list of alkalizing foods. *Outside the body*, lemon juice is acidic (its pH is below 7). Everyone knows this—it's a citrus fruit. *Inside the body*, however, when it has been fully metabolized and its minerals are in the bloodstream, its effect is alkalizing, and it therefore raises the pH of the body. You will also notice that there are some acidifying foods, which I ask you to limit, but which you are allowed to eat freely in the DETOX and ATTACK phase. Again, it's all about balance.

WHAT IS THE IDEAL BALANCE?

The ideal meal should consist of two-thirds alkalizing foods and one-third acidifying foods. I am not asking you to constantly monitor what you are eating to reach the perfect balance. This would become counterproductive and a source of anxiety (which we are trying to avoid!). Finding this balance will become easier after a few days of incorporating more and more alkalizing foods into your diet.

Take the time to have a hard look at your plate, your friends' plates, even, and, this is most revealing of all, other people's shopping carts at the supermarket checkout. You will realize that we usually do the opposite, with one-third alkalizing foods and two-thirds acidifying. Together, we are going to reverse this trend. The menus and recipes at the end of this chapter (p. 306) are specially designed to help your body reach the correct pH balance.

FIVE STEPS TO A HEALTHY, ALKALINE DIET

*a*S WELL as aiming for the right balance of acidifying and alkalizing foods, there are eating habits that you can adopt to improve your diet. Follow these guidelines *for life* and you'll also help to balance your pH.

1. Pass on the salt! As we know, salt is increasingly used in ready meals as a taste enhancer. It's far too easy to get too much of it, which can cause an acidic pH, cardiovascular problems, water retention, and so on. Limit your sodium consumption by cooking without salt and only adding it before serving or eating. Do not leave the salt shaker on the table—keep it far away from the hand and far from the plate. Herbs, spices, and other seasonings make ideal substitutes that will titillate your taste buds without added calories and sodium and, hence, without any impact on your health.

Continued . . .

2. Go raw! How many raw vegetables did you tuck into last week? Include raw fruits and veggies in your meals as often as you can. When I travel to France and to the UK, I often meet with BootCampers who tell me that uncooked vegetables make them feel bloated and give them an intolerable level of gas. This is most likely because they are consumed on an irregular basis. To avoid bloating, abdominal pain, or cramping, it is critical to change your habits slowly. Just like a vegan would be afflicted by stomach pains should she switch to a meat-based diet over-night, a person who eats very few raw foods would suffer if her diet was changed abruptly.

Start with one serving a day, then two, then three, then more, at your own pace, so that your body has time to get used to this new way of eating.

If you did not eat raw foods at all before this program, you will need about six weeks to get to the optimal level of raw food without suffering undue pain and bloating. If you were already eating some, you will need less time to adjust. I aim for eight servings a day of raw food: six of dark, leafy greens or crucifer-ous or sulfur-rich veggies like artichoke and asparagus; and two servings of berries or citrus.

3. Skip the processed food! Thanks to the food-manufactur-ing industry and its colossal marketing budgets, we consume more and more refined products (ready meals, cakes, cookies, fizzy drinks, white bread, white rice, pasta, and so on). But these foods and drinks have undergone so much processing that they have a negative impact on the body's pH.

The vast majority of breakfast cereals contain so much sugar that they are actually unhealthy. A classic breakfast of orange juice from a carton plus a bowl of cereal and milk (containing lactose, a sugar), represents a mega sugar-bomb right at the start of the day. Examine your choices: Go for whole foods, and alternate your glucids (bread, rice, pasta, buckwheat, quinoa) with legumes (lentils, chickpeas, edamame beans), all of which are richer in alkalizing elements, fiber, and minerals.

4. Eat your veggies! Our animal protein intake has greatly increased over the past few decades, replacing healthier vegan protein. This is clear when you think how we plan meals by choosing what will go with the meat or fish, rather than the other way around. Why not start by choosing first which vegetables and whole grains will make the base of your meal and only then decide if you need to add animal protein? If your meal already consists of vegetables or whole grains such as rice or buckwheat, then you can add tofu or legumes as a side dish to obtain the ideal vegan protein balance.

5. The right size! Remember what the size of a portion is, especially when it comes to animal protein (see DETOX, p. 57).

TOP 10 FOODS TO ALKALIZE YOUR DIET

1. LEMON ZEST
Easy to add to your fruit salads and other homemade dishes. Go for organic, unwaxed citrus so you're not ingesting pesticides (remember, they are toxic for our body) and other chemicals.

2. SPROUTED HAZELNUTS
You'll be familiar with my recipe for homemade Hazelnut Milk (p. 71) from the DETOX phase. The great news is that this nut is also wonderful for regulating your pH. Hazelnuts are rich in energy, so don't eat more than fifteen for a snack with an apple, for example.

3. AVOCADO
Stay away from serving avocado with mayo; it's way too rich. Instead, enjoy half an avocado in a veggie sandwich or in a salmon tortilla.

Continued . . .

4. FRUIT AT EVERY MEAL

You already start your day with fresh lemon juice. Now you can add a banana to your breakfast, make a colorful fruit salad for lunch, and round off dinner with a berry crumble.

5. VEGGIES: BRING THEM CENTER STAGE

Steamed artichokes with soy-based mayo; eggplant au gratin; steamed broccoli with a dash of olive oil and a pinch of sea salt; a red cabbage salad or mashed sweet potatoes—these are all easy-to-make dishes that will help you increase your pH, and don't have to be relegated to the side. Use the frozen versions of these vegetables to speed up the cooking process, any time of the year.

6. SPROUTED SEEDS AND GRAINS

Sprouts are highly alkalizing, and are becoming easier and easier to find. Simply top your salads with a few sprouts and, voilà! If you would rather make them yourself, here's a simple method. You don't need any dedicated equipment (though you might find seed-sprouters in health food stores or online). Begin with lentils, quinoa, or alfalfa. Place the seeds or grains in a sieve above your kitchen sink. Each time you go through your kitchen, water them. After a few days (or a few hours, for quinoa) you will have the pleasure of seeing baby sprouts peeking out.

7. ONIONS, SHALLOTS, GARLIC, AND HERBS

Commonly found all year round, these staples will spice up your meals while increasing your pH. Bake a garlic head and serve it with roasted chicken or zucchini au gratin . . . scrumptious! Add shallots to a vinaigrette and raise the culinary bar. Throw fragrant herbs into a simple salad and raise it to the next level. Add chives to a cauliflower purée; rosemary to a ratatouille; bay leaf to a potato gratin, and your dishes will go from "normal" to exotic and chic.

8. SOY AND TOFU

Replace dairy milk with plain soy milk in recipes that call for the real thing and you will be amazed how delicious the dish tastes.

Marinate cubed, firm tofu in equal parts of olive oil, reduced-sodium soy sauce, Dijon mustard, and balsamic vinegar. Stir-fry them—and I guarantee your kids will love it. My teenage son always asks me, "When are you making your Dijon tofu again?" Edamame beans—like in Japanese restaurants—are also great as an appetizer.

9. CINNAMON AND RAW HONEY

Yum! A little bit of honey on a cubed apple over which you sprinkle some cinnamon; or a small coconut-milk yogurt with cinnamon—pure delight! Choose organic raw honey (avoid honey heated to a very high temperature).

10. POTATOES

And you thought that to lose weight you had to banish potatoes from your diet? Not in the least!

Just like lemons, potatoes are acidic outside the body, but alkaline-forming when ingested. (Baked potatoes, with the skin, are the most alkaline-forming. However, almost all commercial, fast-food chips are acidifying.) They are also rich in potassium and calcium.

I am not saying you should tuck them into every meal but if you love your roots then go for it: purple, blue, and red. Try different types to discover new tastes and get the maximum amount of antioxidants (red or blue have the highest levels).

FITNESS TO STABILIZE YOUR WEIGHT LOSS

During ATTACK, we learned to diversify our exercise routine (you may have tried out Zumba classes, aquabiking, Tae Bo, kickboxing, Bokwa, Pilates, yogalates, and so on) because variety does wonders when one is trying to lose weight.

During the MAINTENANCE phase, however, you should find what works for you and stick to it. Studies have shown that you shouldn't be chopping and changing your exercise plan with something new every week. Now is the time to make choices, establish a regular routine you can enjoy, and make it an integral part of your lifestyle. Of course, there is no harm in trying out new sports or exercise classes once in a while, but not with the same magnitude you might have followed when you were in the ATTACK phase.

To maintain your new figure and even go a bit further, we are going to put in place a well-rounded fitness regimen that will keep you motivated. Determine your fitness level (beginner, intermediate, or advanced) and commit to your exercise plan. It is so easy to find "good" excuses not to work out: the kids need to be picked up from school; you have reached your perfect weight and can squeeze into your ideal clothes size; you are too busy with work; your boss has set a tight deadline for a new project; you're home too late or leave too early in the morning.

We women always seem to have too much on our plate (no pun intended) and neglect to place ourselves at the top of our priority list. To be able to love and take care of others, it's essential that you look after yourself. I assure you a good dose of personal TLC will go a long way. So, no more excuses. Carve out time for yourself. I know it might be annoying to be told, "If there's a will there's a way," but it's the truth! I do realize that this will be easier for some, but we can always find a way to do at least something.

FOUR MORE 25TH-HOUR EXERCISES

My "25th-hour" exercises are easy, breezy routines that you can squeeze into a packed routine without even breaking a sweat. We have already learned a few of them in DETOX (pp. 42–46). Here are four new ones:

THE LITTLE RED MAN

Waiting to cross the street? Don't waste this precious time! Standing straight, put all your weight on the right leg, bending the left one slightly and resting on the toes of your left foot. Discreetly push down your left heel while contracting your glutes. Repeat until it burns and then switch legs. If you don't have time to work the second leg, just do it at the next crossing!

THE MOULIN ROUGE SECRET TO A
FIRM DERRIÈRE

A friend of mine who was a dancer at the famous Moulin Rouge cabaret in Paris shared this secret with me. Those ladies are required to display an exceptionally pert behind on stage. My friend told me that she never, ever, rested on her bottom without contracting it. Her theory is not scientifically proven (I state this clearly to avoid scrutiny from fitness professionals), but she claims that if we don't engage our glutes while we rest, we'll get a saggy bum—and we don't want that, do we?

IRON ADDUCTORS

Adductors are the muscles that run down the inner thighs, and you know how hard it is to tone them. I really dislike seeing my inner thighs flabby so I created this easy exercise, which you can perform in bed. Lie on your back, arms along your body, legs straight and together. Open and close your legs as quickly as possible, pointing your toes. Put more thought in the "closing" movement to really engage your adductors. Visualize squeezing a big balloon as you bring them together. Aim for 50 reps per day to get visible results after one month.

STRONG UPPER ARMS

Hold a large (full) bottle of water in one hand, palm facing up, elbow tucked into your side, forearm straight ahead of you and parallel to the ground. Keep your back straight. Without moving your elbow, lower the bottle all the way down and raise it back up. To avoid injuring your elbow, do not overextend your arm. Repeat 20 times and change arms.

THREE MAINTENANCE
FITNESS PLANS

These plans are designed for three progressive levels: beginners, intermediate, and advanced. If you are starting at the first level, do keep up with the pace. Move to the next program once you feel the routine is no longer challenging you. You will shape yourself all the way up to advanced within a few months.

The one-hour walks can be taken during the day in chunks, if that's easier for you than walking the full extent in one go.

A selection of exercises follow the plans. You can vary the program by swapping one exercise for another similar one from this book—for example, you could try Gazelle Legs (page 150) in place of Leg Balancer—but stick to the same duration for each day.

You should also keep fitting in as many 25th-hour exercises as possible.

To see me perform the exercises described throughout the book please go to my blog, valerieorsoni.com, in the Fitness section.

BEGINNERS

MONDAY
30-minute walk on empty stomach, steady pace; plus Butterfly Abs (50 reps); plus 30-minute walk (ramble in the woods or the park, along the river, or on the beach); plus 5-minute Metaboost #1.

TUESDAY
30-minute walk on empty stomach, steady pace; plus the Balancer (50 reps); plus 30-minute walk; plus 5-minute Metaboost #1.

WEDNESDAY
30-minute walk on empty stomach, steady pace; plus Butterfly Abs (50 reps); plus 30-minute walk; plus 5-minute Metaboost #1; plus 20 minutes of fitness exercises (such as Zumba, BodyPump, strength-training, Doggy Paddle).

THURSDAY
30-minute walk on empty stomach, steady pace; plus the Balancer (50 reps); plus 30-minute walk; plus 5-minute Metaboost #1.

FRIDAY
30-minute walk on empty stomach, steady pace; plus Butterfly Abs

(50 reps); plus 30-minute walk; plus 5-minute Metaboost #1;
plus 20 minutes of fitness exercises, as above.

SATURDAY
30-minute walk on empty stomach, steady pace; plus the Balancer
or Butterfly Abs (50 reps); plus 30-minute walk (who said shopping wasn't a sport?); plus one cardio session (bike ride with
friends, for example); plus 5-minute Metaboost #1.

SUNDAY
30-minute walk on an empty stomach, steady pace; plus the Balancer
or Butterfly Abs (50 reps); plus 30-minute walk; plus 5-minute
Metaboost #1; plus 30 minutes of fitness exercises, as above.

INTERMEDIATE

MONDAY
30-minute brisk walk on empty stomach; plus Butterfly Abs (100
reps); plus one-hour walk; plus the Balancer (100 reps); plus 20
minutes of toning exercises: Wall Press-Ups, 45-degree Triceps,
Leg Balancer, Doggy Paddle.

TUESDAY
30-minute brisk walk on empty stomach; plus the Balancer (100
reps); plus one-hour walk; plus Butterfly Abs (100 reps); plus
10-minute Metaboost #2.

WEDNESDAY
30-minute brisk walk on empty stomach; plus Butterfly Abs (100
reps); plus one-hour walk; plus the Balancer (100 reps); plus
10-minute Metaboost #2.

THURSDAY
30-minute brisk walk on empty stomach; plus the Balancer (100
reps); plus one-hour walk; plus Butterfly Abs (100 reps); plus
10-minute Metaboost #2.

30-minute brisk walk on empty stomach; plus Butterfly Abs (100 reps); plus one-hour walk; plus the Balancer (100 reps); plus 10-minute Metaboost #2.

SATURDAY

30-minute brisk walk on empty stomach; plus Butterfly Abs or the Balancer (200 reps); plus one-hour walk (window-shopping counts); plus one cardio session (a long bike ride with the family, spin class, running); plus 10-minute Metaboost #2.

SUNDAY

30-minute brisk walk on empty stomach; plus Butterfly Abs or the Balancer (200 reps); plus one-hour walk (a hike in the woods, along the beach or the river); plus 20-minute fitness session, with exercises of your choice.

ADVANCED

MONDAY

45-minute brisk walk on empty stomach; plus Butterfly Abs (150 reps); plus Wall Press-Ups (20 reps); plus one-hour walk; plus the Balancer (100 reps); plus 20 minutes of fitness and toning (Wall Press-Ups, 45-Degree Triceps, Leg Balancer, Vendetta Hammer).

TUESDAY

45-minute brisk walk on empty stomach; plus the Balancer (150 reps); plus Wall Press-Ups (20 reps); plus one-hour walk; plus Butterfly Abs (100 reps); plus 15-minute Metaboost #3; plus one cardio session.

WEDNESDAY

45-minute brisk walk on empty stomach; plus Butterfly Abs (150 reps); plus Wall Press-Ups (20 reps); plus one-hour walk; plus the Balancer (100 reps); plus 20 minutes of fitness and toning (Reverse Triceps, Leg Balancer, Vendetta Hammer); plus 15-minute Metaboost #3.

THURSDAY

45-minute brisk walk on empty stomach; plus the Balancer (150 reps); plus Wall Press-Ups (20 reps); plus one-hour walk; plus Butterfly Abs (100 reps); plus 15-minute Metaboost #3.

FRIDAY

45-minute brisk walk on empty stomach; plus Butterfly Abs (150 reps); plus Wall Press-Ups (20 reps); plus one-hour walk; plus 15-minute Metaboost #4; plus the Balancer (100 reps); plus one cardio session (Zumba or running).

SATURDAY

45-minute brisk walk on empty stomach; plus the Balancer (250 reps); plus Wall Press-Ups (20 reps); plus one-hour walk; plus one cardio session; plus 15-minute Metaboost #3.

SUNDAY

45-minute brisk walk on empty stomach; plus Butterfly Abs or the Balancer (250 reps); plus one-hour walk (hike); plus 20-minute fitness session with exercises of your choice.

ABDOMINALS

Butterfly Abs ▶

This exercise allows you to work your deep abs and get a flat and sexy tummy. Do this according to your program—and, if you have time, increase to at least four times a week. More is good!

1. Sit comfortably on a gym mat or carpet with your legs in a diamond shape, with the soles of your feet touching. Don't worry if you aren't very flexible at the start. As you progress your knees will eventually reach the ground so that you create the perfect butterfly.
2. Lie down and place your hands under the nape of your neck. Inhale through your nose.

3. Raise your chest about one-third inch while exhaling through your mouth (not forcefully).

4. Lower your chest to the starting position as you inhale, then exhale as you go back up again.

5. Repeat 25 times and, as you progress, up to 50 times. Yes, you can do it!

> ▶ **CAUTION**: Do not push your head with your hands, as this puts your neck at risk of injury. The purpose of your hands is only to keep your head in alignment with your back and shoulders. You don't want to curve your back like a turtle!

The Balancer ▶

For those who want a real challenge to tackle those deep abs, here is the absolute weapon. The Balancer is what we call a "functional" exercise, because it uses the weight of the body (and a small nudge in the right direction with a medicine ball) to strengthen your muscles. You really have to keep your balance with this one!

You can do this anywhere: in your living room during commercial breaks, in the morning after your walk, or in the evening before going to sleep. You are the boss! I recommend you do this exercise once a day (which means going the extra mile, if your program doesn't specify it). It takes 2 minutes and the results are visible almost immediately!

1. If you have fragile knees like I do, I advise you to kneel upright on a gym mat, two beach towels, a carpet, or rug.

2. Keep your back straight.

3. Take a medicine ball or full water bottle and hold it in front of you at chest level with arms slightly bent.

4. Keeping your stomach in, and your arms very slightly bent so as not to put pressure on the elbows, start from the right side and bring the ball down to hip level, around, and up to the left in a semicircular motion. Then, in a controlled manner, bring the ball from the left side down and back to the right. This constitutes one rep.

Beginners: 2-pound weights; 3 series of 10 reps; 15-second rest between series.

Intermediate: 6½-pound weights; 3 series of 30 reps; 15-second rest between series.

Advanced: 13-pound weights; 3 series of 50 reps; 15-second rest between series.

ARMS

Did you know that the shape of our arms can significantly impact how we perceive our body? Toned arms improve the overall body appearance of even a plumper person. As with your abs, toning up your arms doesn't require a superhuman effort or spending endless hours at the gym. You can work on your triceps and biceps throughout the day or in just a few minutes in the morning and at night.

Since the forearms are usually toned enough thanks to our daily activities, we won't need to focus on them.

45-Degree Triceps ▷

The triceps are located between your elbow and your shoulder on the back of your arm and are the hardest arm muscles to tone. This exercise is one I particularly love because it is quick, easy, and incredibly efficient.

1. Take two weights (you can use two bottles or two cans of identical weight). Hold your weights in both hands and stand with your feet shoulder-width apart, abs tight. Bend forward from the waist at a 45-degree angle.
2. As you exhale, pull your arms back so that the upper part of your arms is in alignment with your torso, and your elbows are bent. This is the starting position.
3. As you inhale, push the weights back to straighten your arms and feel the contraction in your triceps.
4. Return your arms to the starting position as you exhale.

Beginners: 4-pound weights; 3 series of 20 reps; 15-second rest between series.

Intermediate: 8-pound weights; 4 series of 25 reps; 15-second rest between series.
Advanced: 12-pound weights; 5 series of 30 reps; 15-second rest between series.

TIPS: Be aware of your posture. Don't round or arch your back; keep it as straight as possible when you bend forward. Check your posture in a mirror if you can. Don't forget to breathe!

Wall Press-Ups ▶

If you want to continue working your triceps, do 20 Wall Press-Ups every time you go to the loo. We learned this one in DETOX, but here's a reminder:

1. Stand facing a wall, feet hip-distance apart, close enough to touch it with your arms straight out, at eye level.
2. Place your palms on the wall and bend at the elbows to do 20 standing press-ups.
3. Push your body back from the wall harder each time, moving slowly and maintaining control.

TIP: Increase the difficulty of this exercise by keeping your fingers off the wall, or by working only one arm at a time.

Doggy Paddle ▶

Do this move whenever you hit the pool or beach!

1. Place flippers on your feet.
2. In the water, lie down on your tummy on a board or float.
3. Let your legs simply float on the surface of the water while your arms paddle.

TIP: You know this move is working when you feel the burn in your triceps, *not* your upper back.

Reverse Triceps ▶

You can do this at home using your sofa, your bed, or a bath that's securely bolted in place, or in the park using a bench. After a few weeks you'll have toned, shapely arms and you'll be able to wear sexy, sleeveless dresses without feeling self-conscious.

1. Stand with your back facing the seat or support. Place your hands behind you on the seat, hip-distance apart, and face forward.
2. Walk your legs forward until they are at a 90-degree angle. Keeping your back straight, use the force in your triceps to lower your body until your bum is just below knee level—do not let your body drop too far.
3. Slowly lift your body back up to its original position, controlling your triceps as you do so. Do not bounce. Try and maintain full control throughout.

Beginners: 2 series of 10 reps; 15-second rest between series.
Intermediate: 2 series of 25 reps; 15-second rest between series.
Advanced: 3 series of 50 reps; 15-second rest between series.

CORE AND UPPER BODY

Vendetta Hammer ▶

Do this exercise three times a week or according to your program. It will:

■ Eliminate stress: Simply visualize whatever it is that is causing you stress and pound it out. It really works!
■ Tone your abs and core, namely the abdominal strap and lower back.
■ Strengthen the muscles of your upper body and arms (anterior deltoids). I'll leave you to discover where else you feel the after-effects of the workout most on the following day!

1. Do this exercise outside so as not to hit anything, or in a room where you have enough space around yourself.
2. Take a heavy weight, according to your fitness level and strength (see below). Personally, a 22-pound weight is enough for me for this exercise.
3. Standing with your legs shoulder-width apart, feet and toes pointing forward, knees slightly bent, back straight, and abs contracted (yes, you can do it!), hold the weight in both hands.
4. "Launch" it above your head, maintaining control throughout. Don't throw the weight, but send it up in a controlled movement. Hold on to the weight tightly so that it doesn't slip out of your hands. It is also very important that your back and abs are nice and tight when you do this exercise, because if not, you can actually damage your back.
5. Return to the starting position by gently lowering the weight.

Beginners: 2-pound weight; 1 series of 25 reps; 15-second rest between series.
Intermediate: 10-pound weight; 2 series of 25 reps; 15-second rest between series.
Advanced: 25-pound weight; 3 series of 30 reps; 15-second rest between series.

LEGS

Leg Balancer ▶

This exercise works your abductor and adductor muscles—inner and outer thighs—and will kill those saddlebags. I do this with a chair at home, or whenever I am in a park or anywhere with a bench. There's no need to be wearing any specific sports gear.

1. Stand straight and place your hands on the top of the chair or park bench.

2. Raise your right leg to the right side of your body, pointing your toes.
3. Slowly lower your leg and flex your foot, remaining in control of the movement and without swinging.
4. Don't rest your foot on the ground but continue the movement as you raise your leg up again on the same side.

Beginners: 2 series of 25 reps each side; 30-second rests between series.
Intermediate: 2 series of 50 reps each side; 30-second rest between series.
Advanced: 3 series of 100 reps each side; 30-second rest between series.

TIP: For an added challenge, let go of the bench or chair that you were using to keep your balance!

METABOOSTS:
FOR WHEN LIFE IS TOO HECTIC
TO EXERCISE PROPERLY!

*f*OR THOSE of us who are pressed for time and cannot follow the fitness plans I suggest, here is another way to squeeze in exercise every single day, even if you are traveling or if your day is too hectic for you to do your one hour of cardio or your 10,000 steps. Follow the MetaBoost specified in the program you are following (either Beginner, Intermediate, or Advanced) and always feel free to add extra ones into your day!

1. METABOOST 5 MINUTE (BEGINNER)
1-minute march on the spot (warm up)
1-minute squats (sit in the air—no chair!—with your
   knees bent at a 90-degree angle)
1-minute Wall Press-ups (p. 300)
1-minute Butterfly Abs (p. 297)
1-minute march in place (cool down)

Or

1-minute march on the spot (warm up)

1-minute skipping rope

1-minute Lunges (p. 147)

1-minute side-to-side leaps over a broom on the floor

1-minute march on the spot (cool down)

Or

5-minute power walk around the block

2. METABOOST 10 MINUTE (INTERMEDIATE)

1-minute march on the spot (warm up)

20 Jumping Jacks (p. 44)

20 side-to-side leaps

20 long jumps (jump in front of you as far as possible)

20 side jumps (this time, use a broom and jump over it from right to left and then left to right)

20 series of hopscotch (hop on one leg, then jump on two legs, then hop on the other leg; 20 jumps on each leg)

1-minute regular speed walk

1-minute frog jumps

1-minute power walk (using arms to pump)

1-minute regular speed walk

1-minute relaxed walk (cool down)

Or

10-minute power walk around the block

Or

10 minutes on your stationary bike at home

3. METABOOST 15 MINUTE (ADVANCED)

1-minute march on the spot (warm up)

20 Jumping Jacks (p. 44)

20 side-to-side leaps

1-minute Wall Press-Ups (p. 300)

1-minute abs (your choice)

1-minute march on the spot

20 Jumping Jacks (p. 44)

20 side-to-side leaps

1-minute abs (your choice)

1-minute squats (sit in the air—no chair!—with your knees bent at a 90-degree angle)

4-minute POWER walk (1 minute at normal speed, then 1 minute at a very fast speed, and repeat)

2-minute squats, while walking (walk, stop, squat; repeat)

1-minute "Sun Salutation Pose" (Stand on your mat. As you inhale, raise your arms over your head, keeping your palms together. Exhale and then slowly bend forward, one vertebra at a time, until your hands touch your toes.)

MAINTENANCE MENUS

To help you balance your body pH, I have put together 2 weeks of easy-to-follow menus with 14 alkalizing recipes.

Should you struggle to produce some of the dishes or to find some of the ingredients I mention, just stick to those meals you enjoy preparing. You can repeat them as often as you like. For instance, if you only like one of my breakfast suggestions, then repeat it, as long as doing so is not boring (I like variety but some people prefer routine). In the end, you decide. This phase is more flexible than others, because MAINTENANCE is for life!

And don't forget, even during MAINTENANCE we stick to our weekly TD Day (p. 128) to help keep our body as toxin-free as possible. By the same token, when you have gone overboard and indulged in too much rich food, insert a BOOSTER (p. 249) to kick-start your weight loss.

DAY 1

BREAKFAST

Juice of half a lemon in 8 ounces room-temperature water

1 cup Sobacha (p. 69)

2 Sweet Buckwheat Crêpes (p. 74) with 1 tablespoon Almond
Butter (p. 340)

■ **Feast:** Blueberries or seasonal berries

LUNCH

Mediterranean Wrap (p. 320)

1 peach

4 squares chocolate

SNACK

1 glass Alkalizing Boost (p. 316)

15 hazelnuts, 1 apple, 3 dates

DINNER

■ **Feast:** Greek Cucumber Tzatziki (p. 338)

Salmon steak baked in foil or parchment wrapper with 1
tablespoon olive oil and 1 teaspoon herbs de Provence

5 tablespoons brown rice

1 handful cherries

DAY 2

BREAKFAST

Juice of half a lemon in 8 ounces room-temperature water

1 cup Sobacha (p. 69)

Peanut Butter–Vanilla Buckwheat Smoothie (p. 316)

■ **Feast:** Pink grapefruit

LUNCH

4 small fish tacos

15 corn chips

1 spring mix salad with Garlic Vinaigrette (p. 110)

1 banana

SNACK

1 Gluten-Free Pancake (p. 318) with 1 tablespoon agave syrup

- **Feast:** 1 orange

DINNER

Mock Mash (p. 333)

1 veggie burger

1 Baked Apple (p. 234)

DAY 3

BREAKFAST

Juice of half a lemon in 8 ounces room-temperature water

1 cup Sobacha (p. 69)

1 Sweet Buckwheat Crêpe (p. 74) with a little Strawberry Jam (p. 77) and a pea-size touch of butter

1 Alkalizing Boost (p. 316)

LUNCH

½ melon

- **Feast:** Tofu with Dijon Mustard (p. 93) (or wrap version, just roll this tofu in a wrap without adding any other ingredients)

Baby potatoes sautéed with garlic

1 orange

SNACK

Raspberry-Coconut Smoothie (p. 186)

DINNER

Beef Spring Rolls (p. 323)

1 Asian mixed salad with Garlic Vinaigrette (p. 110)

5 tablespoons brown jasmine rice, cooked according to instructions

1 vegan yogurt with berries

DAY 4

BREAKFAST
Juice of half a lemon in 8 ounces room-temperature water
1 cup Sobacha (p. 69)
1 slice toasted whole wheat bread with cream cheese
1 slice roast ham
■ **Feast:** Seasonal fruit salad sprinkled with cinnamon

LUNCH
Creamy Avocado and White Bean Wrap (p. 320)
1 orange

SNACK
2 tablespoons almond butter
1 banana

DINNER
Eggplant Tarte Tatin (p. 324)
Baby arugula salad with Balsamic Vinaigrette (p. 195)
Strawberry-Cantaloupe Soup (p. 318)

DAY 5

BREAKFAST
Juice of half a lemon in 8 ounces room-temperature water
1 cup Sobacha (p. 69)
1 serving oat porridge with cinnamon and 1 tablespoon honey
1 Purple Milkshake (p. 72)

LUNCH
Corsican Wrap (p. 198)
1 kiwi

SNACK
1 cup V8
Green Olive Tapenade (p. 338) with 15 gluten-free crackers

DINNER

Radicchio salad with Garlic Vinaigrette (p. 110)

Blackened Tilapia (p. 325) with a mix of sweet corn and young potatoes

■ **Feast:** Red berries

DAY 6

BREAKFAST

Juice of half a lemon in 8 ounces room-temperature water

1 cup Sobacha (p. 69)

1 Sweet Buckwheat Crêpe (p. 74) with Almond Butter (p. 340)

■ **Feast:** Papaya or pink grapefruit

LUNCH

Feta and Olive Pasta Salad (p. 85)

■ **Feast:** Spaghetti Squash with Crimini (p. 334)

3 dried figs and 3 lychees

SNACK

Nucela and Chocolate Smoothie (p. 317)

DINNER

Marinated Leeks with Herbs (p. 105)

Turkey a la Dijonnaise (p. 325)

■ **Feast:** Pineapple Carpaccio (p. 235)

DAY 7

BREAKFAST

Juice of half a lemon in 8 ounces room-temperature water

1 cup Sobacha (p. 69)

1 Savory Buckwheat Porridge (p. 77)

3 prunes

LUNCH

Peanut-Tofu Crunchy Wrap (p. 321)

1 tomato sliced with 1 tablespoon olive oil and salt, to taste

1 cup grapes

SNACK

Flat Tummy Boost (p. 317)

DINNER

Beef Kefta (p. 326)

5 tablespoons couscous (cooked according to instructions)

2 Almond Cookies (p. 341)

DAY 8 (Turbo Detox Day)

BREAKFAST

Juice of half a lemon in 8 ounces room-temperature water

1 cup Sobacha (p. 69)

1 Sweet Buckwheat Crêpe (p. 74)

3 tablespoons unsweetened applesauce

1 pink grapefruit

LUNCH

2 gluten-free toasts with hummus

1 large ripe tomato sliced with a drizzle of olive oil and basil

■ **Feast:** Seasonal berries

4 squares chocolate

SNACK

10 raw almonds

■ **Feast:** Papaya Granita (p. 340)

DINNER

Bok Choy with Shrimp (p. 327)

5 tablespoons basmati brown rice

1 banana

DAY 9

BREAKFAST

Juice of half a lemon in 8 ounces room-temperature water

1 cup Sobacha (p. 69)

2 scrambled eggs cooked with 1 tablespoon of
nonhydrogenated margarine

1 slice whole wheat bread, toasted

1 peach

LUNCH

1 cup Creamy Kasha (p. 328)

3 slices turkey deli

■ **Feast:** Strawberries

SNACK

10 hazelnuts

1 coconut milk yogurt

DINNER

Pork Chili Verde (p. 329)

1 small steamed potato, mashed with 1 tablespoon
nonhydrogenated margarine

■ **Feast:** Lychees

DAY 10

BREAKFAST

Juice of half a lemon in 8 ounces room-temperature water

1 cup Sobacha (p. 69)

1 Alkalizing Boost (p. 316)

½ cup unsweetened muesli

1 cup almond milk

LUNCH

Curry Chicken (p. 330)

Mashed steamed broccoli with 1 tablespoon
nonhydrogenated margarine

½ cup gelato (your choice)

SNACK

10 walnuts

2 cups blueberries

4 chocolate squares

DINNER

Belgian Endive Boats with Salmon (p. 331)

½ cup whole wheat orzo drizzled with olive oil and 1 tablespoon Parmesan cheese

1 pink grapefruit

DAY 11

BREAKFAST

Juice of half a lemon in 8 ounces room-temperature water

1 cup Sobacha (p. 69)

1 cup buckwheat porridge cooked in almond milk, topped with 1 tablespoon honey, 1 teaspoon raisins, and 1 tablespoon pine nuts

1 cup raspberries

LUNCH

Turkey Club Wrap (p. 321)

Romaine salad with Garlic Vinaigrette (p. 110)

2 Chocolate Pebbles (p. 342)

SNACK

1 whole wheat pita bread

3 tablespoons Baba Ganoush (p. 339)

DINNER

Cucumber Mousse (p. 335)

1 portion Fish and Shrimp Crumble (p. 262)

½ cup unsweetened applesauce

DAY 12

BREAKFAST

Juice of half a lemon in 8 ounces room-temperature water

1 cup Sobacha (p. 69)

3 store-bought gluten-free waffles

3 slices salmon

½ avocado, mashed

1 orange

LUNCH

Your favorite Indian restaurant:

Vegetarian biryani

Palak paneer

■ **Feast:** Fruit salad

SNACK

10 raw almonds

1 banana

DINNER

Moroccan Carrot Salad (p. 319)

Chicken Piccata (p. 332)

5 tablespoons steamed quinoa

4 squares chocolate (your favorite)

DAY 13

BREAKFAST

Juice of half a lemon in 8 ounces room-temperature water

1 cup Sobacha (p. 69)

1 croissant (let's indulge)

■ **Feast:** Orange

LUNCH

1 cup Hawaiian Rice Salad (p. 319)

2 slices deli turkey

1 handful cherries

SNACK

½ melon

10 walnuts

DINNER

Sautéed Potatoes and Artichokes (p. 336)

1 soy patty

Chocolate Pudding with Coconut Cream (p. 237)

DAY 14

BREAKFAST

Juice of half a lemon in 8 ounces room-temperature water

1 cup Sobacha (p. 69)

1 cup low-fat cottage cheese mixed with 1 tablespoon honey, 3 tablespoons unsweetened muesli, and 2 tablespoons blueberries

LUNCH

Super Gourmand Wrap (p. 322)

Romaine salad with Balsamic Vinaigrette (p. 195)

4 fresh figs

SNACK

1 Flat Tummy Boost (p. 317)

15 hazelnuts

DINNER

Garden salad with Balsamic Vinaigrette (p. 195)

Cabbage Blinis (p. 337) with smoked salmon

1 slice Moist Grapefruit Cake (p. 344)

MAINTENANCE RECIPES

ALKALIZING BOOST

SERVES 1

½ organic cucumber, unpeeled

1 Asian pear, unpeeled

2 slices ginger, peeled

1. Place all the ingredients in your juicer.
2. Serve in a glass and enjoy right away!

PEANUT BUTTER–VANILLA BUCKWHEAT SMOOTHIE

SERVES 1

4 tablespoons steeped buckwheat (after you have made your Sobacha)

1 cup almond milk

1 banana

1 tablespoon peanut butter

1 teaspoon vanilla extract

1. Put all ingredients in a blender and blend until smooth. Enjoy!

NOTE: This can keep for 4 hours in the fridge. The contents will separate; reblend before serving.

NUCELA AND CHOCOLATE SMOOTHIE

The word nucela *comes from the Corsican word for "hazelnuts," a nut that is a staple of the Corsican diet. And it reminds me of a famous hazelnut/chocolate spread brand!*

> 1 cup hazelnut milk (see Note below)
> 1 banana
> 1 teaspoon vanilla extract
> 1 tablespoon raw agave nectar
> 1 tablespoon raw chocolate powder or 85 percent dark chocolate

1. Put all ingredients in blender and blend until smooth. Enjoy right away or store, covered, in the fridge. It can keep 2 days.

   NOTE: You can use store-bought or homemade hazelnut milk from the Hazelnut Milk Smoothie recipe (p. 71).

FLAT TUMMY BOOST

> ¾ cup almond milk
> 2 sprigs fresh mint
> 3 ice cubes
> 1 pinch matcha green tea powder
> 1 packet stevia or 1 teaspoon agave nectar

1. Combine all the ingredients in your blender. Enjoy immediately!

GLUTEN-FREE PANCAKE

SERVES 4

1 cup sweet chestnut flour, sifted

1 cup rice flour, sifted

4 tablespoons finely ground almonds or hazelnuts

2 cups coconut or rice milk

1 teaspoon oil

Pinch salt

1. Combine all the ingredients in a salad bowl. If you find the batter too thick, add up to ¼ cup of water to achieve desired consistency.
2. Heat a pancake griddle to medium heat.
3. Pour in one ladle of batter. Cook over medium heat for 2 to 3 minutes, then turn over and cook on the other side, until slightly brown (indicates doneness).

STRAWBERRY-CANTALOUPE SOUP

SERVES 4

2 small cantaloupe melons, cut in half, seeds removed

1 teaspoon vanilla extract

10 strawberries

10 mint leaves

1. Use a melon-baller to form some melon balls to garnish, then scoop out the rest of the melons.
2. Put the melon flesh in a blender and puree to obtain a smooth consistency. Add the vanilla extract and mix.
3. Pour the soup into a bowl. Cut the strawberries and add them and the melon balls to the soup. Add mint leaves.
4. Refrigerate until ready to serve.

MOROCCAN CARROT SALAD

SERVES 4

1½ pounds young carrots, peeled, julienned

4 tablespoons olive oil

1 teaspoon cumin

Salt and pepper, to taste

1. Bring a pot of water to boil. Steam the carrots with a little salt in a steamer basket set over boiling water for about 10 minutes (any longer and they'll be soggy).
2. Place carrots in a salad bowl and add the olive oil, cumin, salt, and pepper (you can add more cumin according to your preference). Mix well. Let cool before serving.

HAWAIIAN RICE SALAD

SERVES 4

1 cup brown rice

4 cups chicken broth

2 slices fresh pineapple, diced

4 slices baked ham, diced

1 teaspoon honey

4 tablespoons sweet peas (raw or cooked)

4 tablespoons sweet corn (raw or cooked)

1. Cook the rice with the chicken broth according to package instructions, but reduce cooking time slightly so that rice remains al dente.
2. While rice is cooking, heat the pineapple in a nonstick skillet set over medium heat; as soon as some juice is released from the pineapple, add the ham and let cook until the rice is ready.
3. When the rice is cooked, drain it, reserving some of the cooking liquid.
4. Add the rice to the skillet, along with the corn and peas and some of the reserved liquid, scraping the bits from the bottom of the skillet. Stir well.

MEDITERRANEAN WRAP

SERVES 1

1 corn tortilla

2 tablespoons Baba Ganoush (p. 339)

3 tablespoons cooked couscous

2 tablespoons cooked chickpeas

1 cup cooked chicken, chopped

¼ cup feta cheese, crumbled

¼ onion, thinly sliced

½ cup romaine salad, chopped

1 tablespoon vinaigrette

1. Spread Baba Ganoush on wrap.
2. Pile up all other ingredients, drizzling the vinaigrette evenly over all the wrap. Roll and enjoy!

CREAMY AVOCADO AND WHITE BEAN WRAP

SERVES 1

½ avocado, mashed

2 tablespoons soyonnaise

1 tablespoon balsamic vinegar

1 gluten-free wrap

¼ cup cooked white beans

1 tablespoon shredded Parmesan

3 tablespoons sweet corn (raw or cooked)

½ cup baby arugula

1. In a small bowl, combine avocado with soyonnaise. Add vinegar and mix again.
2. Spread avocado mixture on the wrap, add the white beans, the Parmesan, and sweet corn. Add arugula.
3. Roll and enjoy!

PEANUT-TOFU CRUNCHY WRAP

SERVES 1

1 clove garlic, crushed

2 tablespoons Thai peanut sauce

1 whole-wheat wrap

½ cup firm tofu, cubed

½ cup Asian salad mix

2 tablespoons peanuts, crushed

1. Mix garlic with peanut sauce. Spread on wrap. Add tofu cubes, then greens. Add peanuts.
2. Roll and enjoy.

TURKEY CLUB WRAP

SERVES 1

1 tablespoon ketchup

2 tablespoons soyonnaise

1 gluten-free wrap

2 slices deli turkey

1 slice provolone cheese or soy cheese

2 leaves romaine lettuce, chopped

1 tablespoon bacon bits

1. Mix ketchup and soyonnaise. Spread on wrap.
2. Add turkey, provolone cheese, and romaine.
3. Top with bacon bits.
4. Roll and enjoy.

SUPER GOURMAND WRAP

1 whole-wheat wrap

1 tablespoon Dijon mustard

4 tablespoons French pâté (your choice)

10 cornichons, halved

½ cup spring mix salad

Pepper, to taste

1. Spread the mustard on the wrap. Mash pâté over mustard.
2. Spread cornichons evenly.
3. Add salad, season with pepper, and roll.

BEEF SPRING ROLLS

SERVES 5

2 tablespoons olive oil

2 onions, minced

1 pound ground beef

Salt and pepper, to taste

1 tablespoon cumin, or to taste

½ bunch cilantro, chopped

1 pack rice wraps (about 1 pound)

Mint, rice wine vinegar and salad greens for serving

1. In large pan, caramelize the minced onion in olive oil over low heat for about 30 minutes. (Add water if necessary.)
2. Add the ground beef and cook for 15 minutes. Season with salt, pepper, cumin, and cilantro. Set aside and let cool.
3. Place a wrap on a plate. Spoon 1 tablespoon of meat onto the wrap and roll it up like a spring roll. Repeat with the remaining filling and wraps.
4. In a sautéing pan, heat some canola oil and fry the spring rolls until golden brown. Place them on a paper towel to absorb the excess oil.
5. Serve with salad greens, rice wine vinegar to dip the rolls, and fresh mint.

EGGPLANT TARTE TATIN

SERVES 6

2 to 3 eggplants

4 tablespoons olive oil

1 clove garlic

1 lemon, juiced

6 sun-dried tomatoes

3 rosemary sprigs

2 ounces pine nuts

1 teaspoon granulated sugar

1 puff pastry sheet, thawed

Kosher salt and pepper, to taste

1. Rinse, dry, and slice the eggplants (about ½-inch thick). Place slices in a colander, sprinkle with salt, and let sit in colander for about 30 minutes, to draw out excess moisture.
2. After 30 minutes, remove any excess salt and pat dry the eggplant slices.
3. In a skillet, heat the olive oil over medium-high heat. Season eggplant slices with some lemon juice, garlic, salt, and pepper and sear. Remove from heat and set aside to cool.
4. Preheat oven to 350°F. Spray a 12-inch-round cake pan with nonstick cooking spray, and set aside.
5. Coarsely chop the dried tomatoes and rosemary, and set aside.
6. In a small skillet over medium heat, toast the pine nuts until golden.
7. Sprinkle sugar into prepared cake pan. Scatter pine nuts, rosemary, and dried tomatoes over bottom of pan. Arrange the eggplant slices in an overlapping circle.
8. Finish with the puff pastry sheet and delicately poke it with a fork.
9. Bake on middle rack until the dough is golden brown, about 25 minutes.
10. When ready to serve, invert the tarte tatin onto a serving plate.

BLACKENED TILAPIA

SERVES 2

2 fillets tilapia

4 tablespoons Cajun spices

2 tablespoons canola oil

Salt and pepper, to taste

Lemon wedges, for serving

1. Rub fillets with spices. Let sit for 15 minutes so that the flavors penetrate into the flesh.
2. Heat oil in a skillet over medium heat. Sauté the tilapia fillet until cooked and reddish-brown (this is what we call "blackened").
3. Serve right away (this kind of recipe does not keep well) with the lemon wedges.

TURKEY A LA DIJONNAISE

SERVES 2

2 tablespoons canola oil

2 boneless turkey breast halves, skin on

¼ cup dry white wine

4 tablespoons Dijon mustard

1 tablespoon tarragon

Salt and freshly ground black pepper, to taste

1. Heat canola oil on medium heat and sauté the turkey until golden brown and cooked through. Remove from pan and cover to keep warm. In the same pan (do not wash between steps), add the white wine and scrape the brown bits, then add the mustard and the tarragon. Mix well. Season to taste wih salt and pepper.
2. Pour the Dijon sauce over turkey, and enjoy right away.

BEEF KEFTA

This dish can be prepared in advance, in a large batch, which you can freeze for future use.

1 pound lean ground beef

3 tablespoons fresh chopped cilantro

3 tablespoons fresh chopped parsley

2 tablespoons ground cumin

4 pinches hot paprika (or hot pepper)

2 cloves garlic, minced

2 tablespoons olive oil

2 large onions, sliced

6 large tomatoes, minced, juices reserved

Salt and pepper, to taste

1. In a bowl, thoroughly mix the ground beef with 2 tablespoons of cilantro, 2 tablespoons parsley, 1 teaspoon cumin, 2 pinches of paprika, and 1 clove of the minced garlic.
2. Heat the olive oil in a large saucepan (or a tagine pot if you own one) over low heat. Caramelize the onions (this will take 30 minutes). Add the tomatoes and their juices. Let simmer for 20 minutes and add the rest of the cilantro, parsley, cumin, paprika (or hot pepper), and the remaining minced garlic clove. Season with salt and pepper.
3. Roll ground beef mixture into meatballs to form 1½-inch balls. Add them to the saucepan.
4. Cover and cook over low heat for 20 minutes, stirring often. Serve and enjoy!

BOK CHOY WITH SHRIMP

SERVES 4

2 bok choy or Chinese cabbage

½ pound small shrimp, cooked and cut into small pieces

1 apple, diced

Juice of ½ lemon

⅓ bunch fresh cilantro

1 tablespoon sesame seeds (black, preferably, for a nice color effect)

FOR THE VINAIGRETTE:

1 tablespoon soyonnaise

1 tablespoon canola oil

1 tablespoon rice wine vinegar

Salt and pepper, to taste

1. Rinse the bok choy and pat dry. Steam for 5 minutes.
2. Chop and place in a salad bowl. Add the shrimp and apple, and pour the lemon juice over.
3. Add the dressing and mix well.
4. Garnish with the sesame seeds and chopped cilantro.

CREAMY KASHA

½ cup kasha (roasted buckwheat)

4 cups chicken broth

1 tablespoon shredded Parmesan

2 Laughing Cow cheese wedges

Salt and freshly ground black pepper, to taste

1. Cook kasha until tender in chicken broth according to package directions. Drain.
2. Put back into the pot and add the cheeses. Mix well. You should have a creamy texture.
3. Season with salt and pepper.

PORK CHILI VERDE

Tomatillos, referred to as green tomato ("tomate verde") in Mexico, are a staple in Mexican cuisine, and used to make traditional green salsa. The jalapeño chile pepper is now found everywhere in the world. Originally from Mexico, it can be stuffed, preserved in salsa or vinegar, or dried. The poblano chile pepper is relatively large and rather mild. It is generally used fresh or dried; for this recipe, feel free to use other sweet peppers if you cannot find these Mexican peppers.

This is a great dish to make in big batches as it freezes and reheats very well.

¼ cup, plus 2 tablespoons canola oil

4 pounds pork butt or shoulder, trimmed of fat and cut into 2-inch cubes

2 yellow onions, chopped

6 cloves garlic, minced

1 teaspoon salt

Pepper, to taste

1 teaspoon cumin

4 cups chicken stock

4 poblano chiles (fresh, dried, or marinated)

4 jalapeño chiles (fresh, dried, or marinated)

2 yellow peppers, seeded and diced

3 pounds tomatillos

1 bunch cilantro, chopped

1. In a large soup pot, heat ¼ cup of the canola oil over high heat and brown the pork cubes. Remove and set aside.
2. Drain the fat and reduce heat to medium. In the same pot, heat 2 tablespoons of canola oil and sauté the onion and garlic. Season with salt and pepper. Cook until translucent. Add the browned pork. Add cumin and chicken stock, and let mixture simmer for 30 minutes.
3. Combine peppers, tomatillos, and cilantro and purée. Add pepper purée to pork mixture and simmer for an additional 30 minutes.
4. You can serve this dish with brown rice and white beans, just like in Mexico!

CURRY CHICKEN

2 tablespoons canola oil

2 skinless chicken breasts, chopped into medium-size cubes

1 cup canned light coconut milk

2 tablespoons curry

Juice of 1 lime

Salt and freshly ground black pepper, to taste

1. In a skillet, heat canola oil over medium heat and sauté chicken cubes until golden.
2. Add coconut milk, curry, and lime juice. Simmer on low for 5 to 10 minutes until chicken is cooked through.
3. Season with salt and pepper, to taste, and serve.
4. Can be kept in the fridge for up to 3 days, well covered.

BELGIAN ENDIVE BOATS WITH SALMON

The endive belongs to the chicory family and can be served cooked or raw. A vegetable rich in kaempferol—a powerful antioxidant that reduces the risk of cancer in general and has a beneficial effect on certain cancers, endive also reduces the risk of cardiovascular diseases. Enjoy this delightful and nutritious dish!

1 head Belgian endive

1 teaspoon fat-free cream cheese

1 slice smoked salmon

1 teaspoon fish roe, orange or black color

Dill, for serving

1. Rinse and dry the endive leaves. Spoon some cream cheese on each leaf.
2. Using scissors, chop the smoked salmon over the cream cheese. Top with fish roe.
3. Garnish with dill, and serve chilled as an appetizer.

CHICKEN PICCATA

1 lemon

6 chicken breasts, skin removed

Salt and freshly ground black pepper, to taste

½ cup organic whole wheat flour

¼ cup olive oil

1 ounce nonhydrogenated margarine

5 ounces button mushrooms, sliced thinly

1 clove garlic, finely chopped

1 tablespoon tapioca or cornstarch

½ cup dry white wine

1 tablespoon capers

1½ tablespoons sugar

1. Peel the lemon with a sharp knife and remove the membranes. Cut the lemon into pieces, reserving the juice.
2. Season the chicken breasts.
3. Heat ¼ cup oil in a frying pan over medium-high heat. Brown the chicken breasts for 3 to 5 minutes per side. Remove from the pan and set aside.
4. To the hot frying pan, add the nonhydrogenated margarine. Sauté the mushrooms for approximately 2 minutes. Add the garlic, tapioca, and wine. Stir well and bring to a boil.
5. Add the lemon and its juice, capers, sugar, and salt and pepper, to taste.
6. Simmer for a few minutes to allow the sauce to reduce slightly.
7. Pour the sauce over the chicken and serve hot with steamed green beans.

MOCK MASH

What are mock mashed potatoes? They are mashed potatoes made without potato but with cauliflower and cheese. A true delight! Don't hesitate to make extra, because these mashed potatoes freeze very well.

1 head cauliflower, chopped into florets

3 tablespoons nonhydrogenated margarine

4 wedges Laughing Cow cheese or organic equivalent

Salt and pepper, to taste

Nutmeg, to taste

1. Steam the cauliflower in a steamer basket for 20 to 30 minutes until it can be easily mashed with a fork.
2. While mashing, add margarine, cheese, salt, pepper, and nutmeg.

SPAGHETTI SQUASH WITH CREMINI

SERVES 4

I love spaghetti squash. Nature must have had fun creating this hybrid pasta-squash!

1 spaghetti squash, halved lengthwise, seeds removed

5 tablespoons olive oil

1 pound cremini mushrooms, sliced

2 cloves garlic

Salt and freshly ground black pepper, to taste

6 tablespoons grated Swiss cheese, Pecorino, or soy cheese

1. In a large saucepan, place one half of the squash, flesh side down. Cover with water and bring to a boil.
2. Cover and simmer for 20 minutes.
3. In the meantime, heat the olive oil in a sauté pan over medium heat and sear the mushrooms and garlic with some salt until cooked through and crispy.
4. When the spaghetti squash is fork-tender, remove from the pan and set aside to cool. Repeat cooking process with remaining spaghetti squash half.
5. Preheat oven to 375°F.
6. To remove the spaghetti strands from the shell, drag a fork from end to end across the squash (the flesh looks like spaghetti). Be careful to not pierce the shell. Place squash in a bowl and reserve the shells.
7. Add the mushrooms to the squash flesh and season with salt and pepper.
8. Fill the shells with the mixture and sprinkle with grated cheese. Transfer the spaghetti squash to the oven and bake for 20 minutes until nicely browned.

CUCUMBER MOUSSE

SERVES 4

A smooth, light, and alkalizing recipe (remember, cucumber helps you keep a balanced pH).

2 cucumbers

1 ounce fat-free sour cream, or vegan alternative

2 egg whites

Kosher salt and freshly ground black pepper, to taste

Chopped parsley, for garnish

1. Peel and cut the cucumbers in half. Remove the seeds. Place them in a food processor, and pulse to chop. Pass the purée through a fine-mesh strainer.
2. In a bowl, combine the sour cream and the cucumber purée.
3. Beat the egg whites until they are fluffy in texture but not firm and gently fold them into the purée. Season with salt and pepper, and refrigerate for 1 to 2 hours.
4. Sprinkle with chopped parsley and serve with toasted whole wheat pita bread.

SAUTÉED POTATOES AND ARTICHOKES

1 large onion, finely sliced

4 tablespoons olive oil

4 red potatoes

6 ounces artichoke hearts (fresh or frozen), cut into quarters

5 ounces fresh or frozen garden peas

1 clove garlic, minced

6 sprigs thyme

Kosher salt

4 cups chicken stock

1. Heat 2 tablespoons olive oil in a skillet over low heat. Add onions and cook until caramelized, about 30 minutes.

2. In the meantime, par-boil the potatoes (in their skin) in salted water. Remove them before they are fully cooked—they should remain firm and inedible. When the potatoes have cooled, remove their skins and cut potatoes into cubes.

3. Add the potato cubes to the caramelized onions. Add the artichoke hearts and peas.

4. Add the rest of the olive oil to the mixture. Add the garlic and thyme, and season lightly with salt (the chicken stock already contains salt, so be careful not to add too much).

5. As soon as there is no more liquid in the skillet, start adding chicken broth, a little at a time. There is no need to soak the vegetables, but keep them moist. Continue adding broth as needed until the potatoes are fork-tender. Remove from heat and serve hot.

CABBAGE BLINIS

SERVES 6

1 teaspoon juniper berries

1 cabbage, sliced thinly

4 eggs

1 teaspoon cornmeal

Salt and freshly ground black pepper, to taste

1 ounce nonhydrogenated margarine

1. Heat a nonstick frying pan over low-medium heat. Toast the juniper berries for 1 minute. Remove from heat and allow to cool fully, then crush the berries.
2. Steam the cabbage for 10 minutes in a steamer basket—it should stay slightly crunchy. Then let cool.
3. Beat the eggs with the cornmeal, salt, and pepper. Add the cabbage and crushed juniper berries.
4. Melt the margarine in small pan over low heat. Form little pancakes with the batter and cook for 5 to 10 minutes on each side.
5. These blinis can be prepared in advance and warmed in the oven before serving.
6. Serve accompanied by steamed fish or a fresh salad for a light meal!

GREEK CUCUMBER TZATZIKI

SERVES 2

1 cucumber, skin on

2 cloves garlic, crushed

1 bunch mint, thinly minced

1 small bunch cilantro, thinly minced

4 tablespoons olive oil

1 cup sheep's milk yogurt

1 teaspoon salt

Pepper, to taste

1. Grate the cucumber and place in a colander. Add 1 teaspoon salt and let sit for 15 minutes over the sink or a deep dish.
2. Transfer cucumber to a salad bowl, add all other ingredients, and mix well. Put in the fridge for at least 30 minutes. Serve chilled.

GREEN OLIVE TAPENADE

SERVES 1

A recipe from Corsica and Provence that you can enjoy as a dip, add to a salad dressing, or use in a fish en papillote recipe.

7 ounces green olives, pitted

1 tablespoon capers

2 anchovy fillets

1 tablespoon olive oil

Freshly ground black pepper, to taste

1. Chop the olives, capers, and anchovies, and combine in a bowl.
2. Add the olive oil and pepper. If you prefer a less coarse tapenade, pulse the mixture a few times in a food processor.
3. Refrigerate until ready to eat.

BABA GANOUSH

SERVES 6

Here is a nice way to get your RDA in folacin (folic acid) and potassium. The typical American diet lacks these two critical nutrients. Folacin is essential for the manufacture of genetic material as well as protein metabolism and red blood cell formation. Potassium helps maintain regular fluid balance and is necessary for nerve and muscle function.

3 medium-size eggplants

Juice of 1 lemon

5 anchovy fillets (canned, in olive oil) (optional)

Mayonnaise or soyonnaise (optional)

2 cloves garlic

⅓ cup olive oil

1. Poke holes in the eggplants using a fork, and microwave on high for 8 minutes. Cut eggplants in half and scrape the pulp into a food processor.
2. Add the lemon juice, olive oil, anchovy fillets, soyonnaise, and garlic. Pulse until you achieve the desired consistency.
3. Serving suggestion: Serve cold with pita bread, hummus, and a few olives for a Middle Eastern combo plate!

PAPAYA GRANITA

The papaya is sometimes called the "new elixir of youth." Its important content of provitamin A and vitamins C and E are, in fact, a considerable source of antioxidants. It's a small pleasure with the multiple virtues!

1 papaya

5 ice cubes

1 teaspoon vanilla extract

5 tablespoons lime juice

Mint leaves, for garnish

1. Divide the papaya in half. Remove seeds.
2. Scrape the flesh and place in a mixing bowl.
3. Add the ice cubes, lime juice and vanilla, and blend to obtain a thick granita.
4. Pour into a cup and decorate with mint leaves. Enjoy right away!

ALMOND BUTTER

You'll need a high-speed blender for this recipe. If you are buying one, make sure it mentions "nut butters" on its packaging or specifications.

2 cups raw almonds

½ cup orange juice

Dash sea salt

1. In a powerful blender, blend the almonds with ¼ cup orange juice and salt. If mixture is too dry, slowly add remaining ¼ cup juice, to reach desired consistency.
2. Keeps 2 weeks if kept in a jar with a tight lid in the fridge.

ALMOND COOKIES

MAKES 24 COOKIES

½ cup nonhydrogenated margarine, melted

½ cup, plus 2 tablespoons white sugar

1 large egg

1½ cups gluten-free flour

½ envelope baker's yeast

1 cup almonds, crushed coarsely

1 tablespoon orange water

Zest of one lemon

1. Preheat oven to 375°F. Lightly oil a baking sheet and set aside.
2. In a mixing bowl, whisk margarine with sugar. Add egg and mix. Slowly add flour, then the yeast. Mix carefully to form a smooth batter.
3. Add almonds, orange water, and lemon zest. Mix again; the texture should be quite thick.
4. Form small balls of dough and place them on prepared baking sheet leaving 1½ inches between each ball of dough as they will expand as they bake.
5. Cook for 8 to 10 minutes, until golden.

CHOCOLATE PEBBLES

MAKES 25 PEBBLES

You will need a small round cookie cutter or mini cheesecake ring about one-inch in diameter.

> 3 tablespoons coconut oil (be very precise or the shape won't hold when you bake them)
>
> 3 tablespoons brown sugar
>
> 1 egg
>
> 12 ounces plain, gluten-free granola (see Note, below)
>
> 8 ounces baking milk chocolate (fear not, we won't be using all of it! The large quantity makes the coating easier)
>
> 1 tablespoon canola oil

1. Preheat the oven to 340°F. Line a baking sheet with parchment paper and set aside.
2. In a medium bowl, mix the coconut oil, sugar, and egg. Incorporate the granola and mix well.
3. Form your pebbles using the cookie cutter directly on the parchment paper. Spoon some of the mix inside, press well using the end of a spoon, the flat side of a wine bottle cork, or simply your fingers, and remove the mold carefully. Repeat with remaining mixture.
4. Bake for 6 minutes or until the top of the pebbles are golden but not brown. The color changes fast so keep an eye on them (with my oven it is precisely 6 minutes 30 seconds!).
5. Allow pebbles to cool completely, or place in refrigerator to speed things up.
6. Melt the chocolate with the canola oil in a double boiler (a bain-marie for the francophiles).
7. As soon as the chocolate is ready (don't let it sit around, use immediately), coat the pebbles: using tongs, take each pebble one at a time, dip the uneven side in the chocolate, and place it smooth side down on a sheet of wax paper to set. Repeat with remaining pebbles; place in refrigerator to set chocolate coating.

8. Pebbles will keep for up to 5 days in the fridge and will delight your guests at the end of a dinner party or make an amazing treat for the children alongside a juicy autumn apple.

NOTE: You can use regular granola if you aren't gluten intolerant. Also, be sure to use a non-crunchy version, as the "crunchy" nuggets are too large and don't work well in this recipe. My favorite brand is Udi's.

VARIATION: For a coconut version, add 3 tablespoons coconut flakes to the base mix and a little more to decorate the top of the chocolate coating.

MOIST GRAPEFRUIT CAKE

SERVES 6

Grapefruit is an amazing source of antioxidants: vitamin C, provitamin A, and flavonoids, which protect the body from some degenerative diseases and prevent early skin aging. I guarantee you'll love this cake; it simply melts in your mouth!

1 yellow grapefruit, preferably organic (because we use the skin)

½ cup nonhydrogenated margarine, softened

1⅓ cups confectioners' sugar

2 eggs

1 cup gluten-free flour (my favorite brand is Cup4Cup)

1 teaspoon baking powder

2 pink grapefruits, preferably organic

2 tablespoons Cointreau or any orange brandy

1. Preheat oven to 350°F. Grease an 8-inch baking dish and set aside.
2. Juice the yellow grapefruit. Set juice aside. Using a paring knife, remove the yellow grapefruit peel. Blanch the peel for 2 to 3 minutes. When completely blanched, grate the zest.
3. In a standing mixer, cream the softened margarine with 1 cup confectioners' sugar. Add the eggs, flour, baking powder, grapefruit juice, and the zest. Mix until fluffy and smooth.
4. Pour batter into prepared pan and bake for 35 minutes. Set baking dish on a cooling rack. When fully cool, run a knife around the inside of dish to loosen cake, and invert it into a deep dish.
5. Juice 1 pink grapefruit and combine with the remaining confectioners' sugar and orange brandy. Pour this mixture over the cake and let stand for 5 minutes, to allow mixture to absorb into cake. Garnish with some of the remaining pink grapefruit sections and serve.

THE END

Here we are! If you have reached this page it means that you've either:

- Read the entire book and followed the program, *or*
- Skimmed through the pages to get to the conclusion quickly (piece of advice: Go back to the introduction and take the time fully to immerse yourself in the program, starting with the two weeks of DETOX), *or*
- Read the whole book in one go and are now planning when you are going to begin. Please, don't be overwhelmed; go back to the beginning and get started, one day at a time. (Just a hint: The right time is *now!*)

If you are in the first category of readers, take a moment to look back and see how much your lifestyle has changed since we started out on this journey. You should be lighter, feel more energetic, and empowered with new knowledge in all aspects of your life: fitness, nutrition, stress-management, sleep-management, motivation, and more.

Whenever you feel your old habits creep back into your life, don't hesitate to return to the beginning of this book and reprogram your mind and your life. There is no shame in that. The unhealthy habits were accumulated over years—decades, even—so there is always the possibility that we need to go back to the drawing board once in a while, to fully eradicate them.

I would love to hear from you about your victories, your struggles, and the solutions you found within this program; please let me know about your favorite recipes and your favorite tips. I would be delighted to feature you as a VIP BootCamper on my blog (valerieorsoni.com) so that you can make use of your success story by inspiring others. If you are game, drop me an e-mail at valerie@lebootcamp.com. Don't hesitate to share your journey via a blog right from the start—this will help others jump on the healthy lifestyle bandwagon along with you.

In the meantime, I wish you an amazing life!

ACKNOWLEDGMENTS

The thank-you page is always my favorite page in any book. It is usually the first one I read! I simply love seeing how much of a village it takes to produce a comprehensive book like this one.

Anyway, this is where I get to thank all the people who have made this book a reality.

I am going to start with Sara Hecht and Selina Prager, two ladies who have edited my text since day one. This is truly an international team: I'm from Corsica, Sara is from Australia, and Selina is a South African Londoner. One after the other, they have spent countless hours making sure my words are well chosen and the concepts clearly explained. For your time, for your dedication, and for the impressive end result, I thank you from the bottom of my heart!

To Denise Silvestro at Penguin/Berkley: After meeting with you I knew I wanted to work with you! I am thus so thrilled you decided to go along with my project. Your amazing feedback, experience, and contributions have helped shape up the book. Word by word, line by line, you made sure my writings would be understandable to all. Denise, you took a gold nugget and chiseled it into a lovely jewel! And, I should add, you spent a lot of time in your kitchen testing my recipes! You are such a food lover!

To my nutrition experts at LeBootCamp, Gwénaëlle Beau and Marion Bodin: Thank you for answering my urgent requests for new recipes and new menus with wild ingredients in the blink of an eye.

To Laura Zuili, my French agent, who introduced me to my fabulous agent in the United States, Stéphanie Abou in New York.

To my Dad, thank you for all the research you have continued doing for this book and for insisting on some concepts before anybody else had really acknowledged how important they were. I am thankful, too, for all the great recipes you have created for this book.

To my son: Thank you for gracefully handling my "absences" from your life as I was writing and rewriting chapter after chapter, then deleting them and starting from scratch. Seeing your happy smile, knowing that you were doing great in school, then in college made the whole enterprise even more meaningful. In the process you also became vegetarian, but that's another story!

To the man in my life, thank you for making my life so sweet and light; for making sure I get what I need most to move ahead in life: love.

To Mom: Because you are there, every day, any time, wherever I am and for whatever I need. Thank you. You rock, and you are my rock.

To all the BootCampers around the world, who have been with me for so many years. Thank you for your support and for sharing your success with me. Seeing you slim down in a healthy manner has been so rewarding! A special thank-you to the queen of the guinea pigs, on whom I have tried a lot of techniques, Min Jee. Your weight-loss journey is an amazing source of inspiration for thousands of BootCampers!

To Dr. Howard Hack, from Stanford Hospital, for your support and simple explanations of complex body reactions, a big thank-you.

Thank you to my supportive bunch of friends: Danielle, with whom I practice my news fast every Friday; Selina because you are a rock and you represent a long-time strong friendship; Alexia for your fitness expertise and your constant happy mood; Maureen because you are here, always; Paula for your chicken soup prepared with love; Jo for your protection; Carole for your constant support and trust in me and also for the ni-ouniou, but that's another story; Paula, the New Yorker, for your powerful list-making ability.

Thank you to "La Blande," my local French-speaking friends from literally all around the world, and with whom I enjoy food, wines, and jokes every single week around the table of life: Anne-so, Bea, Claire, Florence, Gérald, Isabelle, Kamel, Khalid, Laurent, Mous, Souhila, Xavier.

Thank you also to Heidi, who has discovered who I am, really, and Aaron for taking really cool pictures of me. Finally, thank you to my Dalriada Gaelic instructor, Àdhamh Ò Broin, for helping me clear up my mind with this complex but beautiful language when I was starting to not make any sense at all of cups, ounces, grams, pounds, kilos, stones, and more!

SOME OF MY FAVORITE BRANDS

When we are introduced to new products it's often difficult to decide which specific brand we should buy. Here are some of my favorites:

Agave Nectar: Madhava, Wholesome Sweeteners
Almond Butter: Nutiva, Artisana, Once Again, MaraNatha, Organic Traditions
Almond Meal/Flour: Bob's Red Mill
Almond Milk: Almond Breeze
Buckwheat Flour/Porridge: Bob's Red Mill, VOlifestyle
Buckwheat Frozen Waffles: Nature's Path
Buckwheat, roasted: bulk aisle at Whole Foods; VOlifestyle
Canola Oil: Spectrum (non-GMO)
Cashew Butter: Artisana
Chicken Broth: Pacific
Coconut Milk, canned: Thai Kitchen, Native Forrest
Coconut Milk, fresh: So Delicious, Califia Farms
Coconut Milk Yogurt: So Delicious
Coconut Oil: Nutiva, Nature's Way, Trader Joe's
Coconut Sugar/Crystal: Coconut Secret, Wholesome Sweeteners, Navitas, Big Tree Farms
Crisp Mix for gluten-free crumbles: Among Friends
Gluten-free Baking Mixes: Bob's Red Mill; Among Friends
Gluten-free Bars: Kind (caramel, almond, sea salt is my favorite)
Gluten-free Bread: Schär, Udi's
Gluten-free Crackers: Mary's Gone, Blue Diamond Nut Thins
Gluten-free, dairy-free Frozen Pizzas: Daiya
Gluten-free Granola: Udi's
Hummus: Sabra
Nonhydrogenated Margarine: Earth Balance

Olive Oil, virgin cold-pressed: There are lots of GMO-corrupted olive oils out there. An amazing site to stay on top of your choices is extravirginity.com. Some of my favorite brands are Schiralli, Balduccio, California Olive Branch, Cotsco Kirkland Toscano, O-live (in Canada), Whole Foods California 365, Trader Joe's 100% Greek Kalamata.

Peanut/Almond Butter: Justin's, MaraNatha, Artisana, Nutiva

Raw Bars: Go Raw, Two Moms in the Raw

Raw Chocolate (powder and nibs): Healthworks, Navitas, Viva Labs

Sobacha, ready-made: VOlifestyle

Soyonnaise: Trader Joe's

Stevia: Stevia in the Raw

Vegan Buttery Spread: Earth Balance

Vegan Cheese: Dayia

Water: Voss in glass bottles

YOUR WEIGHT-LOSS PROGRESS PAGE

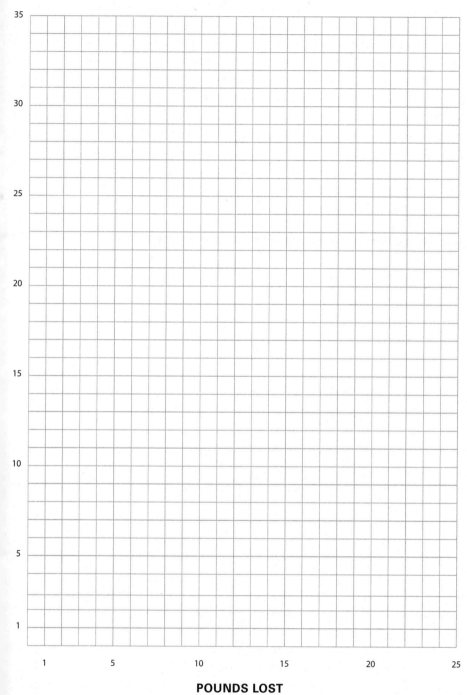

POUNDS LOST

351

REFERENCES

ALKALINE DIET

Dawson-Hughes, B., S. S. Harris, and L. Ceglia. Alkaline diets favor lean tissue mass in older adults. *American Journal of Clinical Nutrition*, 2008; 87(3): 662–665.

Dawson-Hughes, B., S. S. Harris, N. J. Palermo, C. Castaneda-Sceppa, H. M. Rasmussen, and G. E. Dallal. Treatment with potassium bicarbonate lowers calcium excretion and bone resorption in older men and women. *Journal of Clinical Endocrinology and Metabolism*. 2009; 94(1): 96–102.

Frasetto, L., R. C. Morris, Jr., D. E. Sellmeyer, K. Todd, and A. Sebastian. Diet, evolution and aging—the pathophysiologic effects of the post-agricultural inversion of the potassium-to-sodium and base-to-chloride ratios in the human diet. *European Journal of Nutrition*. 2001; 40(5): 200–213.

Reddy, S. T., C. Y. Wang, K. Sakhaee, L. Brinkley, C. Y. Pak. Effect of low-carbohydrate high-protein diets on acid-base balance, stone-forming propensity and calcium metabolism. *American Journal of Kidney Diseases*. 2002; 40(2): 265–274.

Sebastian, A., L. A. Frassetto, D. E. Sellmeyer, R. L. Merrian, and R. C. Morris, Jr. Estimation of the net acid load of the diet of ancestral preagricultural Homo sapiens and their hominid ancestors. *American Journal of Clinical Nutrition*. 2002: 76(6): 1308–1316.

Ströhle, A., A. Hahn, and A. Sebastian. Estimation of the diet-dependent net acid load in 229 worldwide historically studied hunter-gatherer societies. *American Journal of Clinical Nutrition*. 2010; 91(2): 406–412.

DETOX

Dodes, J. E. The amalgam controversy. An evidence-based analysis. *J AM Dent Assoc.* 2001; 132: 348–356.

Duyff, R. L. Healthful eating: the basics. *American Dietetic Association Complete*

Food and Nutrition Guide. 3rd ed. Hoboken, NJ: John Wiley & Sons; 2006: 48.

Eaton, D. C., et al. Renal functions, anatomy, and basic processes. *Vander's Renal Physiology*. 7th ed. New York, NY: the McGraw-Hill Companies; 2009.

Kotkas, L. J. Spontaneous passage of gallstones. *Journal of the Royal Society of Medicine*. Royal Society of Medicine Press; 1985.

Madhus, K. and A. Stromme. Increased excretion of Cs-137 in humans by Prussian blue. *Zeitschrift fur Naturforschung*. 1968; 233b: 391–3.

Nesterenko, V. B., V. I. Babenko, and T. V. Yerkovich. Reducing the 137Cs load in the organism of "Chernobyl" children with apple-pectin. *SMW*. 2004; 134: 24–7.

Position of the American Dietetic Association: Food and nutrition misinformation. *Journal of the American Dietetic Association*. 2006; 106: 601–607.

GLYCEMIC INDEX AND GLYCEMIC LOAD

Foster-Powell, K., S. H. Holt, and J. C. Brand-Miller. International table of glycemic index and glycemic load values. *American Journal of Clinical Nutrition*. 2002; 76: 5–56.

Oregon State University works reviewed by Simin Liu, M.D., M.S., M.P.H., Sc.D. Professor and Director, Program on Genomics and Nutrition, Professor of Epidemiology and Medicine, UCLA School of Public Health. University of Sydney: http://www.glycemicindex.com.

YEAST CONNECTION

Crook, W. G. *The Yeast Connection Handbook*. Jackson, TN: Professional Books, Inc.; 2002.

Crook, W. G. and H. Cass. *The Yeast Connection and Women's Health*. Jackson, TN: Professional Books, Inc.; 2003.

Elmer, G. W., C. M. Surawics, and L. V. McFarland. Biotherapeutic agents, a neglected modality for the treatment and prevention of selected intestinal and vaginal infections. *JAMA*. 1996; 275: 870–76.

Guglielmetti, S., D. Mora, M. Gschwender, K. Popp. Randomized clinical trial: Bifidobacterium bifidum MIMBb75 significantly alleviates irritable bowel syndrome and improves quality of life—a double-blind, placebo-controlled study. *Ailment Pharmacol Ther*. 2011; 33(10): 1123–1132.

Majamaa, H. and E. Isolauri. Probiotics: a novel approach in the management of food allergy. *J Allergy Clin Immunol*. 1997; 99: 179–185.

Nobaek, S., M. L. Johansson, G. Molin, et al. Alteration of intestinal microflora is associated with reduction in abdominal bloating and pain in patients with irritable bowel syndrome. *Am J Gastroenterol.* 2000; 95: 1231–1238.

Rembacken, B. J., A. M. Snelling, P. M. Hawkey, et al. Non-pathogenic *Escherichia coli* versus mesalazine for the treatment of ulcerative colitis: a randomized trial. *Lancet.* 1999; 354: 635–639.

Tubelius, P., V. Stan, A. Zachrisson, et al. Increasing work-place healthiness with the probiotic Lactobacillus reuteri: a randomized, double-blind placebo-controlled study. *Environ Health.* November 7, 2005.

INDEX

Detox phase recipes (cont.)
Carrot-Garlic Purée, 85
Chicken Tandoori, 100–101
Chicken Tortilla Soup, 78–79
Chicken with Lemon and Cumin, 96
Citrus, Kale, and Prawn Salad, 84
Date Smoothie, 73
Feta and Olive Pasta Salad, 85
Flat Tummy Smoothie, 72
French Creamy Carrot Soup (Crème de
  Carottes), 81
Garlic Scallops, 95
Garlic Vinaigrette, 110
Ginger Bok Choy, 106
Grapefruit-Strawberry Mix, 112
Gratineed Scallops, 88–89
Green Morning Boost, 168
Grilled Shrimp with Coconut Milk, 92
Grilled Trout, Corsican Style, 94
Hazelnut-Crusted Trout, 99
Hazelnut Milk Smoothie, 71
Hummus, 111
Lemon Vinaigrette, 110
Marinated Leeks with Herbs, 105
Mariner's Mussels, 102
Parisian Crumble, 114–15
Parmesan-Buckwheat Crêpes, 75
Pink Trout Rillettes, 90–91
Poulet Basquaise, 97
Provençal Stuffed Zucchinis, 108–9
Purple Milkshake, 72
Raita, 86
Raspberry Panna Cotta, 116
Ratatouille Provençale, 103
Red Snapper with Citrus and Fennel
  Salad, 98
Rhubarb and Strawberry Compote, 117
Salmon en Papillote, 87
Savory Buckwheat Porridge, 77
Sobacha, 69
Soup au Pistou, 82–83
Stir-Fried Tofu with Dijon Mustard, 93
Strawberry Jam, 77
Sweet Buckwheat Crêpes, 74
Tri-Color Fruit Salad, 113
Zucchini and Caramelized Onion
  Gratin, 107
Diets. See also LeBootCamp Diet; Toxic
  diets
alkaline-balancing, 287–89
Cabbage Soup Diet, 26
cellulite and, 140
diet foods, 29
dieting, 3

eliminating dairy, 18
fad, 9
high-protein, 26
honeymoon, 127
Lemon Juice/Cayenne Pepper Diet, 26
mono, 26
pH regulation and, 284
Pineapple Diet, 26
during plateaus and benchmarking, 160
saboteurs, 126
2-week detox diet, 46–47
Digestion, 283–84
Diphenyl isatin, 52
Dips
Avocado Dip with Capers, 250, 268
Baba Ganoush, 313, 339
Green Olive Tapenade, 309, 338
Doggy Paddle, 294, 295, 300
Double-blind studies, 4
Dress, 161

Edamame, 251
Honey-Glazed Salmon with Edamame,
  253, 265
steamed, 65
Eggplant Tarte Tatin, 309, 324
Eggs, 23, 46, 53, 108, 247
hard-boiled, 177
Poached Egg with Arugula, 170, 211
Scallion Omelet, 166, 202
scrambled, 176, 179, 311
Enchiladas, 23, 46, 54
Energy vampires, 37, 40, 126
Erythritol, 30, 54
Estrogens, 28
Ethics, 13
Eugenol, 245
European Food Safety Authority, 30
Exercise. See also Bum shaping; Fitness;
  Targeted trouble-zone plan; Tummy
  toning; 25th-hour exercises; Walking
anti-cellulite, 121
bicycle riding, 143, 297, 304
BodyPump, 121, 125, 127, 294
boxer, 146
Butterfly Abs, 294, 295, 296, 297–99,
  303
Doggy Paddle, 294, 295, 300
flat stomach, 44
focused, 12
45-Degree Triceps, 295, 296, 300–301
hiking, 297
Leg Balancer, 296, 302–3
marching, 303, 304

Hazelnut Milk Smoothie, 60, 71, 317
sprouted, 289
Health, 9, 13, 19–20, 25, 35, 157
Healthy Chinese Rice, 175, 226
Hearts of Palm and Chicken Salad, 179, 197
Herbs. *See also specific herbs*
for alkalizing diet, 290
Herb Vinaigrette, 90
Marinated Leeks with Herbs, 61, 105, 310
High-fructose corn syrup (HFCS), 28–29, 54, 248
High-protein diets, 26
Hiking, 297
Hindu prayer, 43
Hollandaise sauce, 23, 46, 54
Honey, 55, 174, 315
for alkalizing diet, 291
Honey-Baked Ham, 181, 219
Honey-Glazed Salmon with Edamame, 253, 265
Hormones, 28, 36
Hummus, 253, 311
in attack phase menus, 167, 170, 176, 180
in detox phase menus, 60, 61, 62
recipe, 111
Hyperoestrogenism, 139

Ideal weight, 19–20
Inner calm, 39
Innovation, 13
Instagram, 9
Intermediate maintenance fitness plan, 295–96
Internal elimination of toxins, 25
Invisible chair, 150–51
Iron abductors, 293
Iron butt, 44
Isothiocyanates, 245

Jenkins, David, 131
Jerusalem artichokes, 55
Caramelized Jerusalem Artichokes, 171, 197
Juicer, 18
Juices. *See also* Lemon juice; Smoothies
Alkalizing Boost, 307, 308, 312, 316
Blue Boost, 58, 70
C-Boost, 250, 254
fruit, 55
Green Morning Boost, 64, 73, 168, 171, 182
Lemon Juice/Cayenne Pepper Diet, 26

Orange Quencher with Mint, 178, 186
vegetable, 175
Watermelon and Strawberry Quencher, 253, 255
Jumping jacks, 44, 304

Kale, 51, 252
Citrus, Kale, and Prawn Salad, 60, 84
Kefir, 244, 249
Ketone bodies, 142
Kidneys, 280–81
Kiwis, 168, 180, 309

LeBootCamp Diet. *See also specific topics*
components, 74
design, 276
double blind studies, 4
following, 140
fundamentals, 277
journey, 122
no deprivation, 57
recommendations, 47
yeast levels and, 243
Leg Balancer, 296, 302–3
Leg sculpting
abductors targeted, 149
adductors targeted, 149
gazelle legs, 150
invisible chair, 150–51
nutcracker, 149
quadriceps targeted, 150
in targeted trouble-zone plan, 148–51
Legumes, 48, 54, 132, 285
Lemon juice
in attack phase menus, 121, 165, 166, 167, 168, 169, 170, 171, 172, 173, 174, 175, 176, 177, 178, 179, 180, 181, 182
in booster phase menus, 241, 249, 250, 251, 252, 253
candida beating food, 244–45
in detox phase menus, 23, 46, 58, 59, 60, 61, 62, 63, 64, 65, 66
Lemon Juice/Cayenne Pepper Diet, 26
Lemon Vinaigrette, 63, 110, 166, 173, 181, 182, 251, 252
in maintenance phase menus, 273, 307, 308, 309, 310, 311, 312, 313, 314
for pH regulation, 286
Lemon zest, 289
Leptin, 39–40
Liposuction, 140
Little red man, 292–93
Lorentz formula, 19